Legal Aspects of Pain Management

Other books in the **Legal Aspects of Health Care** series:

Legal Aspects of Patient Confidentiality by Bridgit Dimond
Legal Aspects of Consent by Bridgit Dimond

Also by the same author published by Quay Books, a division of Mark Allen Publishing Limited:

Patients' Rights, Responsibilities and the Nurse, second edition
Mental Health (Patients in the Community) Act 1995: An introductory guide

Legal Aspects of
Pain Management

BJN monograph

Legal Aspects of Health Care series

Bridgit Dimond

Quay
Books

Mark Allen
Publishing Ltd

Quay Books Division, Mark Allen Publishing Limited,
Jesses Farm, Snow Hill, Dinton, Wiltshire, SP3 5HN

British Library Cataloguing-in-Publication Data
A catalogue record is available for this book

Printed in the UK by Cromwell Press, Trowbridge, Wiltshire

Contents

Foreword

Pain is perhaps the most feared of all the sensations. It generates fear and despair, breaks the victim in its wake and tortures the onlooker, be that family or friend. Old fears of morphine as a potent and potentially lethal drug gave way in the 1970s to a realisation that the drug was an effective analgesic. When administered orally and titrated up to achieve analgesia, it provides pain relief without shortening life. Yet the abuses became evident in society with addiction, tales of 'double effect' and the murderous intent of Shipman.

Lessons from other countries are important. The legalisation of euthanasia in Holland, until recently not legalised but simply not prosecuted when administered within guidelines, has resulted in a swing back amongst professionals. Awareness of the need for palliative care education and training has increased and doctors are realising that every single patient needs to be able to access good symptom control. As Robert Twycross so often said, 'You do not need to kill the patient to kill the pain'.

The law can seem a blunt instrument when a clinician confronts the myriad of clinical issues in any one patient and tries, sometimes without success, to come to a sound decision in the patient's best interest. We can all learn from the precedents that have made case law. European law is now supplementing this legal framework in England and Wales; it is increasingly shaping the attitudes of society to clinical decision-making processes. Yet lawyers often seem terrifying to clinicians, as if they are ready to pounce on any error to make capital out of it, ignorant of the difficulties and uncertainties the clinician faces, as the law appears to set absolutes that may be open to misinterpretation. Patient autonomy is a phrase much bandied about. Often forgotten is the irrefutable principle that each person is autonomous and the autonomy of one cannot override the autonomy of another within the principles of bio-medical ethics.

The contextual legal framework, within which care is delivered to those who are suffering, highlights why failure to respect the duty of care has severe consequences in law. This book sensitively takes the clinical scenario and explores it, providing references and teaching challenges for discussion. For the next generation of healthcare professionals decisions will become harder, not easier. The Internet, with its information explosion, creates new challenges as patients and their families can access vast mounts of unclassified information; some is based on sound scientific enquiry, some is based on validated human experience. But amongst the 'information' or 'pseudo-information' is much that is simply whim or exploitation of the vulnerable. It is through this minefield that the clinician must steer the person in distress. And, as increasingly difficult decisions are taken, ignorance of the law is no defence.

Ilora G Finlay FRCP, FRCGP
Professor The Baroness Finlay of Llandaff

Preface

In 1987 I was seconded from the then Polytechnic of Wales (now the University of Glamorgan) to work with South Glamorgan Health Authority and during that time acted as patient's representative at the Cardiff Royal Infirmary. During my work there we set up several multidisciplinary brainstorming groups to resolve intractable problems in the hospital. One of these was the difficulties of patients who had come to the Accident and Emergency Department with injuries or conditions which required the examination by doctors from other specialities in the hospital, such as paediatrics, orthopaedics etc. It was the policy that pain relief should not be administered by the A&E staff until the patient had been seen by the specialist doctor. Unfortunately this could involve seriously long waiting times for the patients and the situation was clearly unacceptable. One of the members of the brainstorming group was Ann Taylor, a nurse from the intensive care unit. Subsequently, she developed an interest in pain management and moved from the CRI to the University Hospital of Wales, where she now works in the Department of Anaesthetics and Intensive Care. She initiated an international course for multidisciplinary health professionals in pain management and this has since been developed to Masters degree status with other lecturers involved. Ann's work in this field was subsequently recognised when she was appointed as Welsh Woman of the Year in 1999. It has been my privilege to give the legal input to the course and it has always been evident to me that a book covering the legal aspects of pain management would be a useful adjunct not only to those on the pain management course and other similar courses, but to all those many health professionals from a wide range of specialities who have to deal with many complex legal issues relating to pain management. It should also be of benefit to patient groups and relatives and others involved in palliative care. This book is written for all such people. Because of the variety of their disciplines, the generic term (pain) practitioner will be used, and because the majority are female 'she' and 'her' will be used to denote an individual. Many readers may not be acquainted with basic facts of the legal system and so these are briefly set out in early chapters. It is hoped that the book will provide a succinct, useful basis from which practitioners and others can extend their knowledge of the law for the protection of their patients, their colleagues and themselves. In recognition of the origins of these writings and her significant work in pain management, the book is dedicated to Ann Taylor.

Bridgit Dimond
May, 2002

Acknowledgements

Many people have assisted me in the preparation of this book, particularly those who have participated in the Diploma and Masters Courses in Pain Management run by the Welsh National School of Medicine, with their many questions and concerns about legal issues. In addition, I am considerably indebted to the help of Ann Taylor and her colleagues and to Elizabeth Holden, Carys Evans and Joanne Larkman with their assistance on benefits available to those receiving palliative care and Pat Simpson for her many ideas. As always I am grateful to the constant support and encouragement of Bette Griffiths who once again prepared the index and tables of cases and statutes.

To Ann

1

The legal system

> **Box 1.1: Situation**
>
> June was suffering from multiple sclerosis (MS) and experiencing considerable pain. She learnt from an MS support group that fellow sufferers had successfully used cannabis to control the pain. She was given information about how she could obtain it, but was warned that it was contrary to the law and that she could face imprisonment. She decided to take the risk. Unfortunately, she was caught while making the purchase and she and the drug dealer were arrested. June feels that there should not be a law making it illegal for her to have pain relief and is worried about whether she could be sent to gaol. What is the situation?

What is 'law'?

How was any law created to make an MS sufferer taking cannabis a criminal?

Our laws derive from two principal sources: Acts of Parliament/statutory instruments (known as a statutes or legislation) and decided cases. (See the *Glossary* for further explanations of legal terms.) For further information on all aspects of law covered in the book readers are referred to Dimond (2002) and the other works cited in *Further reading* on *page 145*.

Legislation

Legislation, as well as consisting of Acts of Parliament (approval by the Houses of Commons and Lords and the Queen's signature) would include directives and regulations emanating from the European Community, which we as a member state are required to implement and obey (see below).

Legislation can be primary or secondary. As primary legislation it consists of Acts of Parliament, known as Statutes, which come into force at a date set either in the initial Act of Parliament or a date subsequently fixed by order of a Minister (ie. by statutory instrument). The date of enforcement is often later than the date it is passed by the two Houses of Parliament and signed by the Crown. The statute sometimes gives power to a Minister to enact more detailed laws and this is known as secondary legislation. Statutory instruments which are quoted in the text are an example of this secondary legislation. Referring to the situation in *Box 1.1* it is as a result of legislation, in particular the Misuse of Drugs Act 1971, that the use of cannabis is at the time of writing a criminal offence. There are, however, proposals that private personal use of the drug should not be an offence. The Liberal Democrat party adopted this as a resolution at the spring conference in 2002. If a Bill is introduced into Parliament and has sufficient support, then there could amendments to the Misuse of Drugs Act which legalises the use of cannabis in specified situations, but possibly still retaining the criminal offence of dealing. Following approval by both House of Commons and House of Lords and the Queen's signature, the Bill would become an Act and could be brought into force by statutory instrument on a specified date.

Decided cases

The other main source of law is the decisions of the courts. This source is known as case law, or judge made law or the common law. The courts form a hierarchy and the highest court in this country is the House of Lords. If the House of Lords sets out a specific principle, known as a precedent, then this is binding on all courts in the country, except itself (ie. the House of Lords does not have to follow its own precedents). Following the Hillsborough football disaster, the House of Lords had to rule on whether it was lawful to withdraw artificial feeding from a patient in a persistent vegetative state (*Airedale NHS Trust* v. *Bland* [1993]). It held that artificial feeding for Tony Bland could cease, on the basis that that was in his best interests (this is considered in *Chapter 11*).

Each decision of the courts is reported so that lawyers and judges can refer to the case and the principles it established, known as the ratio decidendi which can be applied to any matters in dispute.

If there is a dispute between a case and a statute the latter would take priority: judges have to follow an Act of Parliament. For example, in the Diane Pretty case (*Chapter 2*), the House of Lords could not overrule the Suicide Act which made it a criminal offence for her husband to assist her to die. Had it thought that the Suicide Act was contrary to the European Convention on Human Rights (see below), then it could have referred it back to Parliament. It did not do this. Parliament can enact legislation which would overrule a principle established in the courts. If June were to be convicted for the offence of possession of cannabis, the judge would have considerable discretion over her punishment from an absolute discharge to imprisonment. The court could not overrule the Act of Parliament making the possession of cannabis illegal.

Human Rights Act 1998

This came into force in England, Wales and Northern Ireland on 2 October, 2000 and on devolution in Scotland. It incorporates the Articles of the European Convention on Human Rights into our laws (*Chapter 2*).

Effect of the European Community

Since the United Kingdom signed the Treaty of Rome in 1972, the UK has become one of the member states of the European Community. The effect of this is that the UK is now subject to the laws made by the Council of Ministers and the European Commission. In addition, secondary legislation of the European Community in the form of regulations is binding on the member states. Directives of the Community must be incorporated by Act of Parliament into the law of each member state. Appeals from UK courts on EC laws can be made to the European Court of Justice in Luxembourg which gives interpretations of the European laws. Their decisions are binding on the Courts of member states.

Criminal laws and civil laws

A major distinction in the law of the United Kingdom is that between criminal laws and civil laws. Criminal law are considered in *Chapter 3* and civil laws in *Chapter 4*. Some acts may be actionable as both a criminal offence and also a civil wrong. For example, in *Chapter 6* the action for trespass to the person is discussed. This action can be brought where treatment is given without the consent of the individual and in the absence of other factors which would be a defence to the action (eg. acting out of necessity). A trespass may also be a criminal act of assault and battery and there could be a prosecution in the criminal courts. It can be seen from this that there is not necessarily a moral difference between a crime and a civil wrong.

Legal personnel

Lawyers in this country are trained as solicitors or barristers. The former in the past have had direct dealings with clients and arranged with barristers (known as Counsel) for the paperwork to be drafted and for representation of the client in court. Now increasingly, solicitors are being trained for advocacy and have rights of presenting a case in court. Eventually this may lead to a single legal profession. They share a common foundation training: either a law degree or success in the Common Professional Examination and then would-be solicitors undertake practical training with a firm of solicitors, and take the Law Society's Part 2 examination, called the Legal Practice Course; while would-be barristers study for the Bar with the Council for Legal Education and are then 'called' to the bar after having dined on a specified number of occasions at one of the Inns of Court to which they must belong. A barrister who wishes to practice must then undertake pupillage where they are attached to a practising barrister. Senior barristers are eligible 'to take silk', ie. they become Queen's Counsel (QC) appointed by the Lord Chancellor. Over recent years there have been considerable changes enabling solicitors to have wider opportunities to speak on behalf of clients in court and recently clients have been permitted to have direct access to a barrister. The likely result of all these developments may in the end be a single profession.

Legal aid and conditional fees

Major changes have been made to the legal aid system under the Access to Justice Act 1999.

Part I of the Act provides for two new schemes, replacing the existing legal aid scheme, to secure the provision of publicly-funded legal services for people who need them. It establishes a **Legal Services Commission** to run the two schemes; and enables the Lord Chancellor to give the Commission orders, directions and guidance about how it should exercise its functions. It requires the Commission to establish, maintain and develop a **Community Legal Service**. The Community Legal Service fund will replace the legal aid fund in civil and family cases. The Commission will also be responsible for a **Criminal Defence Service**, which will replace the current legal aid scheme in criminal cases. The new scheme is intended to ensure that people suspected or accused of a crime are properly represented, while securing better value for money than is possible under the legal aid scheme. The Legal Services Commission will be empowered to secure these services through contracts with lawyers in private practice, or by providing them through salaried defenders (employed directly by the Commission or by non-profit-making organisations established for the purpose).

Part II of the Access to Justice Act 1999 makes changes to facilitate the private funding of litigation. A scheme known as 'no win, no fee' or conditional fee system has been introduced. By this system potential litigants can agree with lawyers' terms on which they will be represented. Insurance cover is taken out to meet the expenses of witnesses and other costs arising in case the action is lost. The 1999 Act amends the law on conditional fee agreements between lawyers and their clients, in particular it allows the additional fees payable to a solicitor in a successful case in a no win no fee agreement, to be recovered from the other side. In a recent court decision the Court of Appeal has agreed that the costs of taking out insurance at a reasonable premium could be recovered from the losing party (*Callery* v. *Gray*; *Russell* v. *Pal Pak Corrugated Ltd*).

It is impossible in a work of this size to deal adequately with the complexities of the legal system and the procedures which are followed. The interested reader is referred to the works in the list of further reading (*p. 145*).

Ethics and law contrasted

One's ethics or moral standards derive from a variety of sources; religion, upbringing, personal experience all lead to a person's ethical values. In any democratic society one would hope that there would be a strong reciprocal relationship between the law and ethics. Therefore, many civil and criminal wrongs would also be regarded as ethically wrong. Inevitably, there are likely to be some gaps. For example, in the situation in *Box 1.1*, June may consider that she is morally right in obtaining cannabis to control her pain. After all, what harm is she causing to anyone? Yet at the present time the Misuse of Drugs Act 1971 and the subsequent regulations makes it a criminal offence.

In this book we are concerned with the law and there can be little discussion of ethical issues. In many of the situations we discuss there is also a moral or ethical perspective and the reader is referred to the reading list for sources on ethics in health care for further discussion.

Codes of practice and conduct

These are not in themselves 'laws'. They do, however, provide guidance for professional practice and could be used in evidence in civil or professional conduct proceedings that reasonable practice has not been followed. This is further discussed in *Chapter 5*.

Application of the law to the situation in *Box 1.1*

As the law stands at present June is guilty of a criminal offence. If she were to plead guilty to the offence it is hoped that any magistrate or judge sentencing her would take into account the mitigating circumstances and it may be that she could be given a conditional discharge.

Questions and exercises

❖ Do you consider that the laws on cannabis should be changed to decriminalise its use?

❖ To what extent do you consider that the criminal law and ethical principles should be identical?

❖ Do you consider that barristers and solicitors should combine in a single legal profession?

❖ Consider your own ethical principles. Are there any circumstances in which they do not accord 100% with the laws in this country?

References

Airedale NHS Trust v. *Bland* [1993] AC 789; [1993] 1 All ER 821

Callery v. *Gray*; *Russell* v. *Pal Pak Corrugated Ltd* The Times Law Report 18 July 2001

Dimond BC (2002) *Legal Aspects of Nursing*. Pearson Education, London

2

Human rights

Introduction

This country was a signatory of the European Convention in 1951 and accepted the articles on human rights. However, the Convention was not incorporated into our law at that time. If a person considered his or her rights had been infringed then he or she would have to take the case to Strasbourg where the European Court of Human Rights was sited and to argue the case there. Parliament has now passed the Human Rights Act 1998. This came into force on 2 October 2000 for England, Wales and Northern Ireland (in Scotland the Act came into force earlier on devolution). The Articles of the European Convention on Human Rights, which is set out in Schedule 1 to the Human Rights Act 1998 can be found in the *Appendix*. The Act:

- requires all public authorities to implement the Articles of the European Convention on Human Rights
- gives a right to anyone who alleges that a public authority has failed to respect those rights to bring an action in the courts of this country

- enables judges who consider that legislation is incompatible with the Articles of the Convention to refer that legislation back to Parliament.

The House of Lords considered the Articles of the European Convention in the case of Diane Pretty (*Regina (Pretty)* v. *Director of Public Prosecutions, Secretary of State for the Home Department*). The facts of the case are set out in *Box 2.2*.

Box 2.2: The case of Diane Pretty

Diane Pretty was a terminally ill and incapacitated person suffering from motor neurone disease. She had minimum movement and was unable to attempt to commit suicide. She wished to die but would require assistance which her husband was prepared to give. She was mentally alert and wished to control the time and manner of her dying so as to avoid the suffering and indignity that she would otherwise have to endure. The husband wished to have an undertaking from the Director of Public Prosecutions (DPP) that were he to aid and abet her suicide, he would not be prosecuted under section 2(1) of the Suicide Act 1961 which makes it a criminal offence to aid and abet a suicide.

It was argued on behalf of Diane Pretty that the provisions of the Suicide Act 1961 were incompatible with the European Convention on Human Rights. Articles 2, 3, 8, 9 and 14 were specifically identified as supporting her case.

Article 2: The right to life

It was argued that Article 2 protected the right to self-determination in relation to issues of life and death. It recognised the individual's right to choose whether or not to live and the state had a positive obligation to protect such a right as it had to protect the right to life.

The House of Lords held that the thrust of the language of Article 2 reflected the sanctity attached to life, affording protection to the right to life and preventing the deliberate taking of life save in narrowly defined circumstances. The Article could not be interpreted as conferring a right to die or to enlist the aid of another in bringing about one's own death. The argument put forward on behalf of Diane Pretty ignored two principles deeply embedded in English law, ie:

❖ The distinction between taking one's own life by one's own act, permissible since suicide ceased to be a crime in 1961 and the taking of life through the intervention of help of a third party which continued to be illegal. This principle was stated by the House of Lords in the Tony Bland case (*Airedale NHS Trust* v. *Bland* [1993]).

❖ The distinction between the cessation of life-saving or prolonging treatment on the one hand and the taking of action lacking medical, therapeutic or palliative justification but intended solely to terminate life on the other hand (*Re J. (a minor) (Wardship: Medical treatment)* [1991]). This distinction proved the rationale for the decisions in Bland .

There was nothing to suggest that these two principles of English law were inconsistent with the rulings in the European Court of Human Rights in Strasbourg.

It was not enough for Mrs Pretty to show that the United Kingdom would not be acting inconsistently with the Convention if it were to permit assisted suicide, she had to go further and establish that the UK was in breach of the Convention by failing to permit it or would be so if it did not permit it. Such a contention was untenable.

Article 3: Prohibition of degrading and inhuman treatment

The House of Lords held that Article 3 required states to respect the physical and human integrity of individuals within their jurisdiction. There was nothing in Article 3 which bore on an individual's right to live or choose not to live. 'Treatment' should not be defined in an unrestricted or extravagant way. It could not be plausibly suggested that the DPP or any other agent of the UK was inflicting the proscribed treatment on Mrs Pretty, whose suffering derived from her cruel disease. By no legitimate process of interpretation could the DPP's refusal of proleptic immunity from prosecution to Mr Pretty, if he committed a crime, be held to fall within the negative prohibition of Article 3.

The House of Lords also held that even if Article 3 was held to apply, there was no arguable breach of the negative prohibition in the Article. It could not be said that the United Kingdom was under a positive obligation to ensure that a competent terminally ill person who wished but was unable to take her own life should be entitled to seek the assistance of another without that other being exposed to the risk of prosecution.

Article 8: Right to respect of private and family life

It was argued on behalf of Mrs Pretty that certain features of her case: her mental competence, the frightening prospect facing her, her willingness to commit suicide if she were able, the imminence of death, the absence of harm to anyone else, the absence of far-reaching implications if her application were granted, and the blanket prohibition of section 2(1) of the Suicide Act which applied without taking account of particular cases, justified her application and were evidence for breach of Article 8.

The House of Lords held that no cases decided in Strasbourg supported her contention and, in fact, her rights under Article 8 were not relevant to the case. Even if this was wrong, infringement was justifiable under Article 8.2. The decriminalising of assisted suicide had been reviewed several times (Criminal Law Revision Committee 14th Report 1980 and the Select Committee of the House of Lords Cmnd 7844 1994) and change was unambiguously opposed. Assisted suicide and consensual killing were unlawful in all Convention countries except the Netherlands, but even there Mr Pretty would be liable if he were to assist Mrs Pretty to take her own life.

Article 9: Freedom of thought

It was claimed for Mrs Pretty that her right to protection of freedom of thought, conscience and religion and the manifestation of religion or belief in worship, teaching, practice or observance had been violated. The House of Lords rejected this argument.

Article 14: Prohibition of discrimination

It was argued on Mrs Pretty's behalf that section 2(1) of the Suicide Act discriminated against those who, like herself, could not take their own lives without assistance because of incapacity. The House of Lords rejected this claim. It held that Strasbourg case decisions held that Article 14 was not autonomous but had effect only in relation to Convention rights. Therefore, if none of the articles cited by Mrs Pretty gave her the right she claimed, then Article 14 would not assist her, even if she were able to establish that the effect of section 2(1) of the Suicide Act was discriminatory. The criminal law could not in any event be criticised as discriminatory because it applied to all.

The Director of Public Prosecutions

The DPP had argued that he had no power to grant the undertaking sought. The power to dispense with and suspend laws and their execution without parliamentary consent was denied to the Crown and its servants by the Bill of Rights 1699. Even if he did have power to give the undertaking sought he would have been very wrong to have done so here. He had no means of investigating the assertions made on her behalf, he had had no information at all concerning the means proposed for ending her life. No medical supervision was proposed. It would be a gross dereliction of the DPP's duty and a gross abuse of his power had he ventured to undertake that a crime yet to be committed would not lead to prosecution. The claim against him had to fail on that ground alone.

Outcome following the House of Lords case

Mr and Mrs Pretty were clearly disappointed with the decision by the House of Lords and took their case to the European Court of Human Rights in Strasbourg. On 29 April 2002 the European Court of Human Rights in Strasbourg ruled that the UK Suicide Act (*Chapter 11*) which made it a criminal offence to aid and abet a suicide was not contrary to the European Convention on Human Rights (Gibb, 2002). The Court stated that:

To seek to build into the law an exemption for those judged to be incapable of committing suicide would seriously undermine the protection of life, which the 1961 Suicide Act was intended to safeguard and greatly increase the risk of abuse.

Applying the Human Rights Convention to Jane's situation

Many of the arguments used on behalf of Diane Pretty could also be used on behalf of June, yet probably with the same defeat. She might argue that since cannabis could relieve her pain, then the law making possession of cannabis a criminal offence is causing her to suffer inhuman and degrading treatment and punishment. Against this it could be argued that it is not the state which is causing her pain; it is her own illness and there are other ways of controlling the pain, other than the use of illegal substances. There has not to the author's knowledge been a case where a human rights argument has been success-fully used in court to justify committing the offence of the possession of unlawful substances. However, the possibility that private use of cannabis may eventually be lawful may remedy June's situation. The judge has considerable discretion in sentencing to take account of any mitigating circumstances.

Conclusion

The second of October, 2000 was feared by many NHS trusts, health professionals and lawyers as leading to an avalanche of claims and law suits but like the millennium bug in the field of computers, this has not happened. What appears to have happened is that many litigants are adding a 'human rights' argument to their litigation. A claim for compensation for negligence may be supported by arguing 'and in addition Article 3 of the Convention has been breached'. In general the courts have taken a conservative attitude to the Human Rights Act 1998. However, there have been many successful cases and undoubtedly it is one of the most important and significant pieces of legislation of the last century in the UK. Even when human rights violation claims are defeated in the UK courts, the claimant can still apply to Strasbourg as the case of Mrs Pretty shows (although, as seen above, she lost).

Legal issues relating to a hospital or community-wide pain management service are considered in *Chapter 17*.

References

Airedale NHS Trust v. *Bland* [1993] AC 789; [1993] 1 All ER 821

Gibb F (2002) Diane Pretty loses battle for right to assisted suicide. *The Times*, 30 April

Re J. (a minor) (Wardship: Medical treatment) [1991] Fam 33

Regina (Pretty) v. *Director of Public Prosecutions, Secretary of State for the Home Department intervening* The Times Law Report 5 December 2001

3

Criminal law

Box 3.1: Situation

Alsana was a staff nurse in a district general hospital. Her husband had a chronic back pain condition which the doctor had been unsatisfactorily treating for many years. She took home some controlled drugs to see if they would help him and discovered that they bought considerable comfort. She continued taking these drugs from the cupboard over several months until the theft was discovered. She is now being prosecuted.

What is a crime?

These are laws which mostly derive from statutes, which create offences which can be followed by criminal proceedings in the form of a prosecution. An example of a statutory provision giving rise to criminal proceedings is the Misuse of Drugs Act 1971 which creates specific criminal offences in relation to controlled drugs which are divided into different schedules for the purpose of the criminal laws.

An example of case law which gives rise to criminal proceedings is the definition of murder which was set out in a case in the seventeenth century.

Most of our criminal laws are enforced by prosecutions brought by the Crown Prosecution Service which was created in 1985. Other bodies also have powers to prosecute in specific cases, eg. the Health and Safety Inspectorate, the National Society for the Prevention of Cruelty to Children and Environmental Health Officers. There are other criminal laws such as those created by local authority powers known as by-laws which create local offences. There is also a right of an individual to bring a private prosecution, but this can be costly and of uncertain benefit.

Ingredients of a criminal offence

Whether the criminal offence originates in legislation (eg. the Offences against the Person Act 1861) or case law (such as murder), there are two major elements in the definition of the offence:

- the physical acts — known as the *actus reus*
- the mental element — known as the *mens rea*.

Both elements must be established beyond reasonable doubt in order to secure a conviction.

The *mens rea*, or mental element, includes all those elements which relate to the mind of the accused. The *actus reus* is everything else. There are some crimes where there is no requirement to show a mental element. For example, the sale of medicine by a person who was not qualified and while unsupervised by a pharmacist and which was contrary to section 52 of the Medicines Act 1968 was once held to be a strict liability offence (*Pharmaceutical Society of Great Britain* v. *Logan* [1982]). The law has now been changed. As a rule, however, there is a distaste for offences of strict liability, ie. where there is no requirement for the prosecution to prove *mens rea*.

Criminal hearings

A prosecution is brought in relation to a charge of a criminal offence and heard in the criminal courts where the standard of proof is beyond reasonable doubt. Summary offences are heard in the magistrates court and indictable offences (the more serious offences) in the Crown court, following committal proceedings in the magistrates. Many offences are triable either way and the accused can opt for trial by jury. Currently, there are Home Office plans to extend the number of offences which can only be heard by Magistrates. In the Magistrates court, the Magistrates decide on the facts if guilt has been established and, if so, sentence the accused. They also have the power to commit the accused to the crown court for sentencing by the crown court judge. In the crown court, the jury decide if the accused is guilty and if so the judge sentences the person convicted.

Criminal negligence

Gross negligence in professional practice may amount to the crime of manslaughter. For example, an anaesthetist failed to realise that during an operation a tube had become disconnected as a result of which the patient died. He was prosecuted in the criminal courts and convicted of manslaughter (*R*. v. *Adomako House of Lords* [1994]). There would also be liability on his employers in the civil courts for his negligence in causing the death of the patient. The Law Commission has recommended that the law should be changed to enable it to be made easier for corporations and statutory bodies to be prosecuted for manslaughter and this may lead to more charges being brought in connection with deaths which arise from gross negligence (Law Commission No 237).

Accusatorial system

A feature of the legal system in this country is that it consists of one side with the responsibility of proving that the other side is at fault or guilty, or liable, of the wrong or crime alleged. This is known as an accusatorial system and it applies to both civil and criminal proceedings. In criminal cases the prosecution attempts to show beyond all reasonable doubt that the accused is guilty of the offence with which he is charged. The magistrates, or the jury in the crown court determine whether the prosecution has succeeded in establishing the guilt of the accused, who is presumed innocent until proved guilty. In civil proceedings, the claimant (originally known as the plaintiff), ie. the person bringing the action, has to establish on a balance of probability that there is negligence, trespass, nuisance or whatever civil wrong is alleged. In civil cases (apart from defamation), there is no jury and the judge has the responsibility of determining whether the claimant has succeeded in establishing the civil wrong. The role of the judge or magistrate is to chair the proceedings, intervening where necessary in the interests of justice, and advising on points of law and procedure.

The accusatorial system contrasts with a system of law which is known as inquisitorial where the judge plays a far more active role in determining the outcome. An example of an inquisitorial system in this country is the coroner's court. Here the coroner is responsible for deciding which witnesses would be relevant to the answers to the questions which are placed before him by statute (ie. the identity of the deceased, how, when and where he came to die), and he asks the witnesses questions in court and decides who else can ask questions and what they can ask. As a result of this 'inquisition', he or a jury, if one is used, determine the cause of death.

Application of the law to the situation in *Box 3.1*

Alsana will have to face the consequences of her crime, no matter how noble her objective, this would be taken into account in determining the sentence, not of her guilt or innocence. At the present time she would have the right to elect jury trial. She would face committal proceedings before the magistrates and if committed to the crown court, would plead to the charge. If she pleaded not guilty she would then face a trial before a jury.

Conclusions

There have been several cases where a health professional has been prosecuted in relation to their care of the patient: such as that of Dr Shipman, who was found guilty of the murder of fifteen patients using morphine; Dr Cox who was found guilty of attempted murder when he injected a patient who was in the terminal stages of rheumatoid arthritis with potassium chloride and Dr Bodkin Adams who was found not guilty of killing a patient in an Eastbourne nursing home. These are considered in *Chapter 11*.

Questions and exercises

❖ Do you consider it should remain a right to have jury trial in the crown court for a charge of theft?
❖ What elements do you consider should be taken into account in deciding whether professional misconduct amounts to the crime of manslaughter?
❖ What are the arguments for having a statutory crime of corporate manslaughter?

References

Law Commission No 237 (1996) *Legislating the Criminal Code: Involuntary Manslaughter*. HMSO, London

Pharmaceutical Society of Great Britain v. *Logan* [1982] Crim LR 443

R. v. *Adomako House of Lords* The Times Law Report 4 July 1994

4

Negligence

Civil laws

There are laws (both statutory and case law) which enable citizens to claim remedies against other citizens or organisations as a result of a civil wrong. A large group of civil wrongs are known as torts, of which negligence is the main one, but the group also includes: action for breach of statutory duty, nuisance, and defamation. Actions for breach of contract are not included in the definition of tort. An example of a statute which can give rise to civil action is the Congenital Disabilities Act 1976 which gives a child, who is born alive, the right to sue in respect of negligence which led to him or her suffering from a congenital defect. An example of a case where an application was made to the High Court is that of Diane Pretty (*Chapter 2*). In this chapter we consider the law of negligence and how it applies to pain practitioners.

Elements of a negligence action

A claimant alleging that negligence has occurred and seeking compensation in respect of harm caused by that negligence would have to establish the following elements:

- that a duty of care was owed by the defendant or its employees in relation to the person who has suffered harm
- that there was a reasonably foreseeable breach of this duty
- which caused reasonably foreseeable
- harm which was recognised in law as subject to compensation.

Duty of care

Case law has laid down that a duty of care is owed to those persons who are so directly affected by one's acts that they ought reasonably to be considered as being so affected when the defendant is directing his mind to the acts or omissions which are called in question (*Donoghue* v. *Stevenson* [1932]). However, the law does not require a person to volunteer to assist another, unless there is an existing duty of care. The law does not require a health professional to volunteer to assist at a road accident, though the codes of professional conduct of specific health professionals may require such 'Good Samaritan' acts. (See, for example, the *Code of professional conduct* of the NMC, 2002.)

Breach of the duty of care

In order to establish if there has been a breach of the duty of care it is essential to establish what standard should have been followed. The courts have used, what has become known as the Bolam Test to determine the standard to be expected of a health professional in a specific situation. This derives from the case of *Bolam* v. *Friern Barnet Hospital Management Committee* [1957]. The test was applied in the case of a obstetrician who was alleged to have pulled too long and too hard in a forceps delivery. The House of Lords held that on the facts a breach of the duty of care had not been established and stated as follows (*Whitehouse* v. *Jordan* [1981]):

> *When you get a situation which involves the use of some special skill or competence, then the test as to whether there has been negligence or not is... the standard of the ordinary skilled man exercising and professing to have that special skill. If a surgeon failed to measure up to that in any respect ('clinical judgement' or otherwise) he had been negligent and should be so adjudged.*

Expert evidence is required to establish what would be the reasonable standard of care in the circumstances of the case and whether on the facts that was followed. Experts are required to give 'responsible, reasonable and respectable' opinions relating to the facts of the case (*Bolitho* v. *City and Hackney Health Authority* [1997]) and the recent reforms in civil proceedings following from the report of Lord Woolf recommend that the parties should agree on the experts to give evidence to the court.

Increasingly, guidelines from such bodies as the National Institute of Clinical Excellence and the National Service Frameworks are likely to be incorporated in NHS Trust procedures and protocols setting out the reasonable standard of acceptable clinical practice. There may still be occasions where the specific circumstances of the patient are such that the procedures are not entirely appropriate and so deviations from it are justified. The House of Lords stated in the Maynard case (*Maynard* v. *W. Midlands RHA* [1984]) that:

> *It was not sufficient to establish negligence for the claimant to show that there was a body of competent professional*

opinion that considered that the decision had been wrong if there was also a body of equally competent professional opinion that supported the decision as having been reasonable in the circumstances.

Causation

Failure to establish a causal link between the breach of the duty of care and the harm that was suffered would mean that the claim for compensation would not succeed in court. In one case a child suffering from meningitis was given 300,000 units of penicillin instead of 10,000 units (*Kay* v. *Ayrshire and Arran Health Board* [1987]). The mistake was discovered and remedial action taken. The health authority admitted liability and made an offer to the parents for the additional pain and suffering that the negligence caused the boy. However, the parents argued that the overdose had caused the boy to become deaf and they rejected the board's offer. The House of Lords held that the parents had not established the causal link between the overdose and the deafness and that the boy was not entitled to the larger amount. It is a well-known fact that meningitis itself can cause deafness.

Harm

The claimant must establish that he or she has suffered harm. Harm recognised by the courts as subject to compensation includes personal injury and death and loss or damage to property. Specific rules apply where it is claimed that post traumatic stress has been caused (*McLoughlin* v. *O'Brian* [1982]; *Alcock* v. *Chief Constable of the South Yorkshire Police* [1992]; *White and others* v. *Chief Constable of the South Yorkshire Police and others* [1999]).

Quantum or level of compensation

Occasionally it might be accepted by a defendant that it is liable, but the amount of compensation payable may be disputed. Where a death has occurred, there is a statutory payment of £7,500 known as a bereavement allowance and this would be payable in respect of a person without dependants. Where there are dependants, they could claim for the loss of their dependency.

The headings for compensation include; general damages which cannot easily be calculated in financial terms such as pain suffering, loss of amenity, and special damages, including; sums already paid out and those which can be more closely calculated such as interest, past care, accommodation, future care, claimant's loss of earnings, other future expenses, and education.

Vicarious liability

In practice, the claimant would bring an action against the employer and would have to show that there was negligence caused by an employee who was acting in the course of employment. The employer would then be vicariously liable for the employee's negligence and would have to pay the compensation. Those health practitioners who are self-employed cannot rely on vicarious liability and would have to have their own insurance cover.

Application of the law to the situation in *Box 4.1*

In a situation such as *Box 4.1* the death would be reported to the coroner and subsequently there may well be criminal investigations to establish whether Mary was guilty of a criminal offence (*Chapter 3*).

If civil proceedings were to be brought Mary clearly has a duty of care to her patient; it would appear difficult to argue that a nurse who failed to administer what was correctly prescribed could be anything other than in breach of the duty of care she owed to the patient. The boy's parents would also have to show that the death occurred as a result of the breach of duty of care by Mary. A postmortem may be required to establish if there was causation between the overdose and the death. It is unlikely that Mary would have to pay compensation herself, since her employer would be vicariously liable for her negligence. There is a legal right of indemnity by the employer against a negligent employee to recover the compensation paid out, but an NHS trust is unlikely to claim this indemnity from Mary successfully.

The future

In spite of the significant reforms introduced by Lord Woolf in civil proceedings, bringing a claim for compensation in the civil courts is still seen as a slow, expensive and cumbersome procedure. In addition, the cost of litigation to the NHS is climbing and shows no signs of decreasing. In 2001 a recent report of the National Audit Office stated that the NHS must make provision for outstanding claims of £2.6 billion, together with an estimated liability of a further £1.3 billion where negligent episodes are likely to have occurred, but where claims have not yet been received. The report noted that the number and value of claims continues to rise, and that they are taking on average about five and a half years to settle. Somewhat startlingly, it was found that nearly half the claims settled in 1999–2000 cost more in legal and other costs than the settlement itself. For settlements of up to £50,000, the costs of reaching the settlement are greater than damages awarded in over 65% of the cases (Dimond, 2001). In the light of this report, the Department of Health (DoH) has proposed a new compensation scheme (DoH, 2001). A white paper is to be published in

2002 which may recommend that a new statutory scheme for civil compensation is adopted which includes no fault liability, mediation, a tariff for the amount of compensation payable and structured settlements for the larger payments.

Questions and exercises

❖ What are you views on the introduction of a no-fault liability scheme for negligence in healthcare?

❖ Do you consider that the employer's right of indemnity against the negligent employee should be exercised in the NHS?

❖ How do you think that mediation would work in claims for compensation for clinical negligence?

References

Alcock v. *Chief Constable South Yorkshire Police* [1992] 2 AC 310 HL

Bolam v. *Friern Barnet HMC* [1957] 2 All ER 118

Bolitho v. *City and Hackney Health Authority* [1997] 3 WLR 115

Department of Health (2001) *Press release 2001/03. New Clinical Compensation Scheme for the NHS*. DoH, London: 20 July

Dimond B (2001) Litigation in the NHS: Recommendations for change. *Br J Midwif* **9**(7): 443–6

Donoghue v. *Stevenson* [1932] AC 562

Kay v. *Ayrshire and Arran Health Board* [1987] 2 All ER 417

Maynard v. *W. Midlands RHA* [1984] 1 WLR 634

McLoughlin v. *O'Brian* [1982] 2 All ER 298

National Audit Office (2001) *Handling clinical negligence claims in England. Report of the Controller and Auditor General House of Commons Session 2000–2001.* National Audit Office, London: 3 May

White and others v. *Chief Constable of the South Yorkshire Police and others* [1999] 1 All ER 1

Whitehouse v. *Jordan* [1981] 1 All ER 267

5

Professional registration

Box 5.1: Situation

Chris, a physiotherapist specialising in back disorders was caring for a patient with a chronic back pain. He was manipulating the patient's back when the patient screamed. It was subsequently established that Chris appeared to have caused serious injury to the patient's back. The patient wants to have Chris struck off the state registered list.

Introduction

Significant changes came into effect in April 2002 in respect of nurses, midwives, health visitors and all those professions previously described as 'professions supplementary to medicine'. Two new registration bodies: the Nursing and Midwifery Council (NMC) and the Health Professions Council (HPC) replaced the former United Kingdom Central Council for Nursing, Midwifery and Health Visiting (UKCC) and the Council for the Professions Supplementary to Medicine (CPSM) respectively. Provision is also made in the NHS Reform and Healthcare Professions Bill for the establishment of a Council for the Regulation of Healthcare Professions. This latter body is intended to oversee the operation of the NMC, the HPC and also the General Medical Council (GMC) and the General Dental Council (GDC).

The scope of the professional registration bodies

The main function of the registration bodies is to protect the public by maintaining a register of persons who have been assessed as competent practitioners and ensure that any practitioner whose fitness to practise is brought into question is investigated and, if necessary, a conduct or health committee hearing is held. The ultimate sanction is removal from the register.

NMC and HPC

These organisations were established in April 2002 having existed in shadow form for almost a year before. Their basic functions are laid down in the Health Act 1999 and the detailed rules and regulations which apply to them are set out in statutory instruments (Nursing and Midwifery Order 2001, Statutory Instrument 2002 No 253, Health Professions Order 2001 SI 2002 No 254).

The functions of the NMC and the HPC which under Schedule 3 Paragraph 8(2) of the Health Act 1999 cannot be delegated to any other body are shown in *Box 5.2*.

Box 5.2: Functions of the NMC and HPC

- ❖ Keeping the register of members admitted to practice.
- ❖ Determining the standards of education and training for admission to practice.
- ❖ Giving advice about standards of conduct and performance.
- ❖ Administering procedures (including making rules) relating to misconduct, unfitness to practice and similar matters.

Codes of professional practice

All registration bodies are expected to establish codes of professional conduct for their registered practitioners. These codes are not in themselves law, but breach of the code could be used as evidence in professional misconduct hearings. A new *Code of professional conduct* for nurses, midwives and health visitors was agreed by the UKCC and the shadow NMC prior to the abolition of the UKCC. One of the first actions of the new NMC was to ratify this action and publish the new *Code of professional conduct* for nurses, midwives and health visitors.

Definition of professional misconduct

In the past, health professionals have had a variety of definitions of professional misconduct depending on their specific profession. For example, those practitioners formerly registered with the CPSM could be found guilty of 'infamous conduct', whereas nurses, midwives and health visitors could face professional conduct proceedings for 'conduct unworthy of a nurse, midwife or health visitor'.

The move towards uniformity of the role of the health registration bodies and the establishment of the Council of the Regulation of Healthcare Professions is likely to lead to a uniform definition of professional misconduct across all health professions.

Progress of a complaint

The complaint would be reported to the Investigating Committee of the HPC. This is one of the statutory committees which the Health Professions Council is required to establish and they are known as

Practice Committees. The others are the Conduct and Competence Committee and the Health Committee.

The Health Professions Order Article 22 applies where an allegation is made against a registered person to the effect that:

a)   his fitness to practice is impaired by reason of:

    (i)   misconduct

    (ii)   lack of competence

    (iii)   a conviction or caution in the UK for a criminal offence; or a conviction elsewhere for an offence, which if committed in England and Wales, would constitute a criminal offence

    (iv)   his physical or mental health, or

    (v)   a determination by a body in the UK responsible under any enactment for the regulation of a health or social care profession to the effect that he is unfit to practise that profession, or a determination by a licensing body elsewhere to the same effect;

b)   an entry in the register relating to him has been fraudulently procured or incorrectly made.

A procedure is laid down for dealing with such allegations. Where an allegation is made under 1(b) the Council must refer it to the Investigating Committee. All other allegations are to be referred to screeners or a Practice Committee. Screeners are to be appointed by rules made by Council and can be members of the Council or its Committees, other than a Practice Committee.

Articles 23 and 24 cover the function and appointment of screeners.

Under Article 26 the Investigating Committee shall investigate any allegation referred under Article 22 or 24. The procedure to be followed is set out.

Article 27 sets out the procedure to be followed by the Conduct and Competence Committee. After consultation with the other Practice Committees, the Conduct and Competence Committee shall

a)   advise the Council on:

     (i)   the performance of the Council's functions in relation to standards of conduct, performance and ethics expected of registered professionals.

     (ii)   requirements as to good character and good health to be met by registrants and prospective registrants, and

     (iii) the protection of the public from persons whose fitness to practise is impaired and

b)   consider:

     (i)   any allegation referred to it by the Council, screeners, the Investigating Committee or the Health Committee and

     (ii)   any application for restoration referred to it by the Registrar.

Under Article 28 the Health Committee shall consider any allegation referred to it by the Council, screeners, the Investigating Committee or the Conduct and Competence Committee and any application for restoration referred to it by the Registrar.

Article 29 sets out the procedure to be followed by the Health Committee and the Conduct and Competence Committee.

Article 31 covers interim orders which can be made by a Practice Committee to suspend a person's registration in specified circumstances.

Article 32 sets out the procedural rules for an investigation of allegations.

Article 33 covers the provisions for restoration to the register of persons who have been struck off.

Article 34 covers the appointment of legal assessors. Legal

assessors have the general function of giving advice to screeners, the statutory committees or the Registrar on questions of law arising in connection with any matter which the Registrar of the Committee or screeners are considering. Other functions can be given to the legal assessors by rules made by the Council.

Article 35 covers the appointment of medical assessors who are appointed to give advice to the same persons or committees as legal assessors.

Article 36 covers the appointment of registered professionals as registrant assessors with the function of giving advice on professional practice.

Application of the law to the situation in *Box 5.1*

If Chris is employed, his employer may be sued by the patient for its vicarious liability for any harm caused by negligence by Chris (*Chapter 4*). If he is self-employed, he may well face personal action against him. In addition, the patient is indicating that he is to be reported to the HPC. If a complaint were to be made against Chris to the HPC (and a complaint against a nurse, midwife or health visitor would follow a similar path but to the NMC) it would be investigated by the Investigating Committee and the procedure outlined above would be followed. Ultimately, Chris faces the possibility of being removed from the register.

Conclusion

There is every likelihood that following the initial investigation Chris would face a hearing before the Conduct and Competence Committee with the possibility of being struck off from the HPC register. If he were not struck off, the complainant could, if the NHS Reform and Healthcare Professions Bill is enacted, complain to the new Council for the Regulation of Healthcare Professions and seek a further investigation.

These changes to our system of professional registration are so recent that it is too early to decide if they are effective in protecting the public from practitioners who are unfit to practise.

Questions and exercises

❖ To what extent do you consider that the public is adequately protected from practitioners who are not fit to practise?
❖ How do you consider professional misconduct should be defined?
❖ Examine the role of the Council for the Regulation of Healthcare Professions. Do you consider that it will fulfil a useful purpose?

Reference

Nursing and Midwifery Council (2002) *Code of professional conduct.* NMC, London

6

Consent — adults

Box 6.1: Situation

Julius was a Buddhist who led a very spartan and austere life. He was in the terminal stages of cancer of the pancreas and was in acute pain. However, he was refusing any medication for pain relief. He was visited by a Marie Curie nurse from the local hospice who found it difficult to assist him, when he was refusing basic help which she could provide. She wondered if he could be forced to have medication for his pain. She was aware that his family were very distressed on his account.

The law of trespass to the person

Two legal actions can arise in relation to consent. The first is an action for trespass to the person, where there is no consent to the touching of another person or other legal justification, or there has been fraud or duress in obtaining the consent. In this action, harm need not be proved: merely the touching or apprehension of touching. Trespass to the person includes both battery (the actual touching of the person) and assault (the apprehension of the touching). Battery and assault are also criminal offences, but here we are considering them as civil wrongs. The other action which can arise in relation to consent is one of negligence; where the person has not been informed of significant information. In this action the claimant would have to prove that harm has been suffered which would not have been suffered if the information had been given. (This is considered in *Chapter 10*.)

The basic principle of law is that no mentally competent adult person can be treated, whatever the motive of the defendant without their consent or statutory justification (for example, the Mental Health Act 1983). Reference can be made to the author's book on consent to treatment (Dimond, 2002).

Defences to an action for trespass to the person

The main defences to an action for trespass to the person are: consent by a mentally capacitated person; acting out of necessity in respect of a mentally incapacitated person and statutory justification such as the Mental Health Act 1983. In this chapter consent will be considered; acting on behalf of a mentally incapacitated person is considered in *Chapter 8*. The law relating to consent and children is considered in *Chapter 7*.

Consent

The main defence to an action for trespass to the person is that the person had given their consent to what would otherwise have been a trespass. The consent must have been given by a mentally competent person, voluntarily without duress or fraud and with the knowledge of what was proposed.

Guidance has been provided by the Department of Health on consent, which can be accessed via the Internet and is intended to be updated on a regular basis (DoH, 2001a).

Evidence of consent

Consent can be given by non-verbal behaviour which implies agreement with the intended action (such as rolling up a sleeve for an injection or blood pressure reading to take place) or by word of mouth or in writing. Clearly, if there is a dispute then consent in writing is the preferred evidence that consent was given, but the signature on the form should not be seen as the consent itself, but evidence, following a process of communication between health professional and patient, that the patient understands what is proposed and is giving his or her consent.

Forms have been issued by the Department of Health as part of its *Good Practice in Consent Implementation Guide* (DoH, 2001b), replacing those issued by the NHS Management Executive in 1990 and updated in 1992. The recommended forms can be used by any health professional and should be in place by April 2002.

Mentally competent adult

To be valid the consent must have been given by a mentally competent adult (for children see *Chapter 7*). Competence is a question of fact and in a case involving a Broadmoor patient, a chronic schizophrenic, who was refusing to have an amputation of his leg (even though he was warned that gangrene had set in and he could die without the amputation), the judge laid down three tests of capacity as follows (*Re C. (adult: Refusal of medical treatment)* [1994]):

1. Could the patient comprehend and retain the necessary information?
2. Was he able to believe it?
3. Was he able to weigh the information, balancing risks and needs, so as to arrive at a choice?

Applying these tests to the Broadmoor patient, the judge decided that the patient did have the mental capacity to refuse and the judge issued an injunction to restrain any person amputating his leg without his consent.

Once it is decided that the patient does have the mental capacity to give or refuse consent then the patient can refuse even life-saving treatment for a good reason, a bad reason or no reason at all (*Re MB. (adult: Medical treatment)* [1997]). The Court of Appeal has laid down guidance for applying to the court if there is a doubt over the mental capacity of the patient who is refusing life-saving treatment (*St George's Healthcare NHS Trust* v. *S.*; *R.* v. *Collins ex parte* [1998]). In the recent case of *Re B.* (2002), the President of the Family Division stated that a mentally competent patient could ask for her ventilator to be switched off and that it was a trespass to her person to treat her without her consent (see *Chapter 11* for further discussion of this case).

Where a competent patient lays down in advance what he or she would not wish to happen at a later time — known as a living will or an advance refusal — then this would be binding on health professionals (*Chapter 9*).

Application of the law to the situation of Julius

The key issue in the situation in *Box 6.1* is the capacity of Julius. If he has the mental capacity then he has the right in law to make his own decisions and can refuse pain relief. Even if this is difficult for his family and his nurse to accept, it is his right. If there is concern as to whether he does have the mental capacity to refuse then an application could be made to court to establish whether he lacks the requisite mental capacity. If he is held to lack mental capacity then treatment could be given to him in his best interests (*Chapter 8*).

Questions and exercises

❖ Do you consider that there should be any exceptions, such as pain relief, which should be made to the right of a mentally competent person to refuse treatment?

❖ Examine your processes of obtaining consent. To what extent do you consider that they are sufficiently vigorous for you to defend an action for trespass to the person?

References

Department of Health (2001a) *Reference Guide to Consent for Examination or Treatment*. Department of Health, London; www.doh.gov.uk/consent

Department of Health (2001b) *Good Practice in consent implementation guide*. DoH, London

Dimond B (2002) *Legal Aspects of Consent*. Quay Books, Mark Allen Publishing Ltd, Salisbury, Wiltshire

Re B. (Consent to treatment: Capacity) The Times Law Report 26 March 2002

Re C. (adult: Refusal of medical treatment) [1994] 1 All ER 819

Re MB. (adult: Medical treatment) [1997] 2 FLR 426

St George's Healthcare NHS Trust v. *S.*; R. v. *Collins ex parte S* [1998] 44 BMLR 160 CA

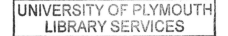

7

Consent — children

Box 7.1: Situation

Avril was twelve years old and was seriously ill with cystic fibrosis. She knew that her lungs were severely damaged following constant chest infections and she had been placed on a list for a lung transplant. She felt that she would prefer to die than put up with the pain, discomfort and suffering and had started refusing her physiotherapy and intravenous antibiotics. Her parents wanted her to continue to have active treatment so that she would be fit for a lung transplant, which could revolutionise her life. What is the law?

Young persons of sixteen and seventeen years

Consent by a sixteen- and seventeen-year-old

These young persons have a statutory right to give consent under the Family Law Reform Act 1969 section 8. Consent can be given for surgical, medical and dental treatment and the definition of treatment covers any procedure undertaken for the purposes of diagnosis and any ancillary procedures such as administration of anaesthetic.

The parents also have the right to give consent on behalf of the sixteen and seventeen-year-old. This is preserved by section 8(3) of the Family Law Reform Act 1969. Where there is a clash between the parent and the minor, the professional would normally follow the wishes of the minor. However, much depends upon the circumstances.

Refusal by a sixteen- and seventeen-year-old

In the case of *Re W.* [1992], a sixteen-year-old, who suffered from anorexia, refused to go to a specialist unit for treatment and the courts decided that she could be compelled to go against her wishes since it was in her best interests to receive treatment. The Court of Appeal held that the refusal of a minor should only be overruled in extreme circumstances where it was a life and death matter. However, this decision was made before the Human Rights Act 1998 became part of English law on 2 October 2000 (*Chapter 2*; *Appendix*). It could be argued that failure to recognise the right of a young person to refuse treatment was a breach of Article 3 and his or her right not to be treated in an inhuman or degrading way. If, for example, W. had been a Jehovah's Witness and had refused blood in a life-saving situation, then to overrule the refusal could have been seen as a violation of Article 3 and also Article 9 (freedom of thought, religion and practice). The point has yet to be considered by the House of Lords.

A mentally incapacitated sixteen- and seventeen-year-old

In the case of *Re B.* the House of Lords laid down the principles for decision making on behalf of a mentally incapacitated seventeen-year-old girl (*Box 7.2*).

> **Box 7.2: Case *Re B. (a minor) (Wardship: Sterilisation)* [1987] 2 All ER 206**
>
> A seventeen-year-old girl (who became later known as Jeanette) who had a mental age of five or six years was in the care of the local authority. It was established that she would have no idea of sexual intercourse, pregnancy and birth. The local authority applied for her to be made a ward of court and for leave to be given for the operation of sterilisation to be carried out.

The House of Lords held that the paramount consideration for the exercise of its wardship jurisdiction was the welfare and best interests of the child. The Court held that it was in the best interests of the minor for the sterilisation to proceed and permission was given for the operation to take place.

The child under sixteen years

While children under sixteen years of age do not have a statutory right to consent to treatment, the right to give consent at common law (ie. judge-made law) was recognised by the House of Lords in the Gillick case (*Gillick* v. *W. Norfolk and Wisbech Area Health Authority* [1986]).

If a child has the maturity to understand the nature, purpose, and likely effects of any proposed treatment, then she could give a valid consent without the involvement of the parents. While the Gillick case itself was concerned with family planning and treatment, the principle applies to other forms of treatment and to boys as well as girls. The principle that the ascertainable wishes and feelings of the child concerned (considered in the light of his age and understanding) should also be taken into account is also stated in the Children Act 1989 section 1(3)(a) as one of the factors to which the court shall have regard in determining what if any orders should be made or varied.

Parents can also give consent to treatment on behalf of their children up to the age of eighteen years. Such treatment must be in the best interests of the child. Persons who do not have parental responsibilities also have power under the Children Act 1989. Section 3(5) enables a person who:

a)   does not have parental responsibility for a particular child; but

b)   has care of the child

to do what is reasonable in all the circumstances of the case for the purposes of safeguarding or promoting the child's welfare.

Parental refusal to give consent

If the parent or guardian of a minor under the age of eighteen refused to give consent to treatment which was necessary in the best interests of the minor, the doctor could act out of necessity in the best interests of the minor according to the principle set out in Re F. (*Chapter 8*). Alternatively, the authority of the court could be sought for treatment to proceed against the parents' wishes. Should the parents fail to give consent to essential treatment or arrange for the treatment to take place, they can face prosecution in the event of harm befalling the child. For example, a Rastafarian couple who had refused on religious grounds to allow their diabetic daughter who was nine years old to be given insulin were convicted of manslaughter on 28 October 1993 in Nottingham. The father was given a sentence of imprisonment and the mother a suspended sentence (*The Times*, 1993).

Application of the law to the situation in *Box 7.1*

Avril is twelve years old and refusing life-saving treatment. While she does not believe that she is likely to survive and receive a transplant, her parents clearly see this as a realistic possibility. Much depends upon her prognosis. It may be that she has become so ill, that she would not have the physical capacity to survive a transplant operation. In this case it may well be in her best interests to be given palliative care to relieve her pain and discomfort but not active interventions. Such a decision needs to be discussed by the multidisciplinary team and Avril's parents and also, according to her mental capacity, Avril could be involved in the discussions. There will be situations where a child of even quite a young age has the mental capacity to understand the prognosis and take an active role in the decisions to be made. Ultimately, if Avril does not have the mental capacity to make the decision, then the doctors caring for her would have to determine, in the light of her prognosis what was in her best interests. In the event of a dispute between parents and clinicians, there would be a referral to court. There are very few cases where the courts have supported parents against the clinicians. In one case (*Re C.* [1997]) parents refused to give consent to a liver transplant being carried out on their toddler. The Court of Appeal held that in the very specific circumstances of the case (the parents lived abroad and as health professionals they believed the transplant not to be in the best interests of the child) the transplant would not be ordered against their wishes.

Questions and exercises

❖ What criteria would you use to decide if a young child had the capacity to give consent to treatment?
❖ In what circumstances do you consider that a young person of sixteen or seventeen should be able to refuse life-saving treatment?
❖ In what circumstances do you consider that a parent should have the power to overrule a refusal to have necessary treatment by the child?

References

Gillick v. W. *Norfolk and Wisbech Area Health Authority* [1986] 1 AC 112
Re B. (a minor) (Wardship: Sterilisation) [1987] 2 All ER 206
Re C. (a minor) (Medical treatment: refusal of parental consent) [1997] 8 Med LR 166 CA
Re W. (a minor) (Medical treatment) [1992] 4 All ER 627
Staff reporter (1993) Insulin ban parents kill their daughter. *The Times*: 29 October

8

Consent — mentally incapacitated adults

Box 8.1: Situation

Julie suffers from Alzheimer's and is in the terminal stages of lung cancer. She is intermittently competent and extremely aggressive towards her carers. She has been transferred from her family home where her daughter was caring for her to a hospice. The staff are uncertain of the extent to which they can compel her to have her medication, some of which is for pain relief.

Introduction

In *Chapter 6* the law relating to consent by a mentally capacitated adult was considered and it was stated that if a person had the mental capacity to make decisions on treatment, then they could refuse even life-saving treatment (*Re MB.* [1997]). This chapter considers the law relating to mentally incapacitated adults.

The mentally incapacitated adult

At the present time no person has the power in law to give consent on behalf of a mentally incapacitated adult. In such a situation the House of Lords has held that professionals have to act in the best interests of such a person (*Re F.* v. *West Berkshire Health Authority* [1989]) and follow the reasonable standard of care as laid down in the Bolam Test.

This principle was laid down in a case involving the sterilisation of a woman with learning disabilities.

The facts are shown in *Box 8.2*.

Box 8.2: Case *Re F.* [1989]

A severely mentally impaired woman had formed an attachment with a fellow patient in a hospital for the mentally handicapped. It was clear that she did not have the capacity to understand or cope with a pregnancy and it was considered that it would be advisable if she were sterilised. However, since she was over eighteen, no one had in law the right to give consent on her behalf.

The House of Lords issued the declaration that she could be sterilised. In giving the required declaration, the court recommended that while most day-to-day activities by professionals on behalf of mentally incapacitated adults could take place under the doctrine of necessity, it wished applications in relation to sterilisations to come before the courts and a Practice Direction covering this was subsequently published.

Best interests

What is meant by the best interests of the patient? This term was discussed in a case where a sister suffering from leukaemia wished to check her elder sister's (referred to here as Y.) compatibility with her prior to the latter providing a bone marrow transplant. Y. suffered both severe physical and mental disabilities and was incapable of giving a valid consent to the blood test or transplant. The court was asked to make a declaration that the blood test and bone marrow could be taken. The court had to decide if this would be in the best interests of Y., not the best interests of the younger sister. The judge argued as follows:

❖ If the sister did not have the bone marrow transplant she would die. This would be a devastating blow to her mother, who suffered from ill health. They were a very close family. The mother would find it more difficult to visit Y. in the community home, especially as after the death of Y.'s sister, she would then have to look after her only grandchild. Y. would suffer as a result of the lack of contact with her mother. The risk of harm to Y. from the blood tests was negligible. Although a general anaesthetic posed some risk, it was a low risk. She had already had a general anaesthetic for a hysterectomy without any apparent adverse ill effects. The bone marrow would regenerate. It was to Y.'s emotional, psychological and social benefit for her to be a donor. It would therefore be in the best interests of Y. for her to have the blood tests and be a donor for her sister.

The declaration that a blood test and, if appropriate, bone marrow harvesting could be taken was therefore issued.

Law Commission proposals

The absence of statutory provisions for decision making on behalf of mentally incapacitated adults and instead reliance on common law powers to act in the best interests of the mentally incapacitated person is unsatisfactory. In the early 1990s the Law Commission carried out extensive consultation to determine what statutory provisions should be made and in 1995 published its proposals, which included a mental incapacity bill at the end of its report. In 1997 a new consultation document was issued by the Lord Chancellor's office and this was followed by a white paper setting out the Government's proposals for decision making on behalf of mentally incapacitated adults. At the time of writing legislation to implement these proposals is still awaited. In Scotland, an Adults with Incapacity (Scotland) Act 2000 came into force in April 2001.

The Law Commission and best interests

The Law Commission recommended that a modified definition of best interests should be used in interpreting the words 'best interests'. It stated that in deciding what is in a person's best interests, regard should be had to:

1. The ascertainable past and present wishes and feelings of the person concerned, and the factors that person would consider if able to do so.
2. The need to permit and encourage the person to participate, or to improve his or her ability to participate, as fully as possible in anything done for and any decision affecting him or her.
3. The views of other people whom it is appropriate and practicable to consult about the person's wishes and feelings and what would be in his or her best interests.
4. Whether the purpose for which any action or decision is required can be as effectively achieved in a manner less restrictive of the person's freedom of action.

Application of the law to the situation in *Box 8.1*

Even though Julie is occasionally mentally incapacitated, it would seem that generally she is unaware of her physical condition and the reason why she is requiring medication. Action needs to be taken in her best interests to ensure that she is receiving pain relief and other care and treatment. Her carers have a power, recognised at common law (ie. the decision of the House of Lords in *Re F.*, see above) to act in her best interests without her consent and follow the reasonable standard of care according to the Bolam Test (*Chapter 4*). Minimum restraint to ensure that she takes the medication could be used in her best interests. Alternatively, there may be justification for her protection in detaining her under the Mental Health Act 1983 to ensure that she receives treatment for her mental disorder.

Conclusion

The absence of statutory provision for decision making on behalf of the mentally incapacitated adult is frustrating for carers, since the common law power is uncertain in its extent and in the use of compulsion. Statutory provision would enable carers in a case such as Julie's to have legal certainty on the extent of their powers and clear procedures to follow for seeking the advice of the court. If of course Julie had, when competent, drawn up a living will which applied to her present situation, then her carers would have been bound to follow that. It is to living wills or advance directives that we turn in the next chapter.

Questions and exercises

❖ At present, relatives do not have the right to make treatment decisions on behalf of a mentally incapacitated adult. To what extent do you consider that this should be changed?

❖ How do you think that best interests should be defined when making decisions on behalf of mentally incapacitated adults?

❖ Do you consider that a mentally incapacitated adult should be given the opportunity of altruistic decisions being made on his or her behalf (such as bone marrow or blood donation)?

References

Law Commission Mental Incapacity (1995) Report No 231. HMSO, London

Lord Chancellor's office (1997) *Lord Chancellor — Who Decides? Decision making on behalf of the mentally incapacitated adult.* The Stationery Office, London

Lord Chancellor's office (1999) *Lord Chancellor Making Decisions. The Government's proposals for decision making on behalf of the mentally incapacitated adult.* The Stationery Office, London

Re MB. (adult: Medical treatment) [1997] 2 FLR 426

Re F. v. *West Berkshire HA* [1989] 2 All ER 545

Y. (adult patient) (Transplant: bone marrow) (1996) 35 BMLR 111; (1996) 4 Med LR 204

9

Living wills

Box 9.1: Situation

Jane's mother had died of Huntingdon's Chorea and when Jane discovered that she too was suffering from the same disease, she drew up, while still mentally competent a living will, stating that if she lost her mental capacity she would not wish to receive any active intervention to keep her alive and this instruction also included direct oral nutrition and hydration. Her living will was signed by her and also witnessed. Three years later it was apparent that Jane was losing her mental capacity and Jane's daughter brought the living will to the attention of the medical and nursing staff caring for Jane. What is the legal validity of her advance directions?

Introduction

As we saw in *Chapter 6*, the treatment decisions of an adult with mental capacity are binding on health professionals. To ignore the refusal to have treatment by a mentally capacitated adult, even if treatment is necessary to save a person's life, is a trespass to the person. This principle also applies to a decision made in advance by a person who is competent at the time of the decision, which is intended to apply at a future time when that person no longer has the mental competence. Such a declaration is known as an advance directive or advance refusal or living will.

Common law validity

The principle that an advance statement of refusal is binding derives at present, not from an Act of Parliament, but from the common law (ie. judge made or case law). In the case concerning Tony Bland who was in a persistent vegetative state following the Hillsborough stadium disaster, the House of Lords had to decide whether his artificial feeding could be stopped (*Airedale NHS Trust* v. *Bland* [1993]). During its deliberations it stated that had Tony Bland, when competent, drawn up a living will to cover that situation, then the health professionals would have been bound by it. A person is completely at liberty to decline to undergo treatment, even if the result of his doing so will be that he will die. This refusal can be declared in advance.

Statutory proposals

The Law Commission in its report in 1995 recommended that advance refusals of treatment should be placed on a statutory footing. This recommendation was rejected in the Government's proposals for decision making on behalf of mentally incapacitated adults. The White Paper in 1999 (Lord Chancellor's office, 1999) stated that:

> *It considered that in the light of the wide range of views on this complex and sensitive subject (ie. advance statements) and given the flexibility inherent in developing case law, the Government believes that it would not be appropriate to legislate at the present time and thus fix the statutory position once and for all. In rejecting the need for a statute covering living wills, the Government stated (paragraph 16) for the clarity of lawyers, doctors and patients what it perceives to be the present position in law.*

The current law and medical practice is as follows. It is a principle of law and medical practice that all adults have the right to consent to or refuse medical treatment. Advance statements are a means for patients to exercise that right by anticipating a time when they may lose the capacity to make or communicate a decision.

Paragraphs 17 to 20 expand on this statement by making it clear that if the advance statement requests specific treatments this does not legally bind a health professional to act contrary to his or her professional judgement. Advance statements do not permit euthanasia 'which is and will remain illegal'.

Essential elements in a living will

The British Medical Association (BMA) has provided guidance in a code of practice on advance directives (BMA, 1995) and this has been specifically commended by the Law Commission (1995) and by the Government (Lord Chancellor's office, 1999). This code of practice sets out the minimum information which should be contained in a living will and recommends the name of a person who could speak on behalf of the person who made the living will being cited. The following information is recommended:

- full name
- address
- name and address of general practitioner
- whether advice was sought from health professionals
- signature
- date drafted and reviewed
- witness signature
- a clear statement of your wishes, either general or specific
- name, address and telephone number of nominated person.

Applying the law to Jane's situation

It has been argued by the author (Dimond, 2000) that the absence of statutory provision can create difficulties and uncertainties for health professionals and Jane's situation, as set out in *Box 8.1*, is an example of one such problem. The Law Commission had recommended that it should not be legally possible for a living will to cover basic nursing care. It defined basic nursing care as including pain relief and direct oral nutrition and hydration. If this proposal had been enacted in a statute, health professionals would have had to interpret Jane's living will as not including oral nutrition and hydration. They would therefore have been justified by statute in continuing to provide that for her. The absence of statutory provision leaves an uncertainty and until there is a court ruling on the issue, health professionals are in a dilemma as to whether they can lawfully withhold food and drink from Jane on the basis of her living will, or continue to insist that she has direct oral nutrition and hydration contrary to its wording.

Resolving the uncertainty

Faced with this dilemma, health professionals would be wise to seek the declaration of the court on the validity of the will and its reference to oral nutrition and hydration.

The High Court in the case of *Re B.* (2002) had to decide if a mentally capacitated woman was able to ask for her ventilator to be switched off. The decision was that a mentally capacitated adult has the right in law to refuse even life-saving treatment and it was a trespass to her person to treat her without her consent (see *Chapter 11* for further discussion of this case).

Future

In the light of such cases as Diane Pretty and *Re B*. it is likely that living wills will become more popular. Clarity by statute as to whether such a document could validly include an advance refusal to have pain relief would be welcomed by those involved in pain management.

Questions and exercises

❖ What arguments are there in favour of drawing up a living will?

❖ Do you consider that health professionals should have any discretion in whether or not the directions in a living will should be followed (eg. in respect of refusal of pain relief or basic nursing care)?

❖ What essential features do you consider should be required for a living will to be legally valid?

References

Airedale NHS Trust v. *Bland* [1993] AC 789; [1993] 1 All ER 821

British Medical Association (1995) *Advance Statements about Medical Treatment*. BMA, London

Dimond B (2000) The legal aspects of living wills: A need for clarity. *Int J Pall Care* **6**(6): 304–7

Law Commission Mental Incapacity (1995) Report No 231. HMSO, London

Lord Chancellor's office (1999) *Lord Chancellor Making Decisions. The Government's proposals for decision making on behalf of the mentally incapacitated adult*. The Stationery Office, London

Re B. (Consent to treatment: Capacity) The Times Law Report 26 March 2002

10

Giving information

Box 10.1: Situation

Mohammed was suffering from severe back pain and sought the advice of an orthopaedic surgeon who advised him that he required surgery to remove a disc which was causing the intractable pain. He was not told that there was a risk of paralysis of the leg if he had this operation. He agreed to the operation and then found that he could not move his left leg. He wishes to sue the surgeon but has been told that the operation was carried out reasonably and there was no negligence in how it was performed. What is his legal situation?

Introduction

In *Chapter 6* it was explained that there were two aspects to the law on consent: the law of trespass and the law of negligence which included the duty of care to inform the patient of significant risks of substantial harm. The law of trespass was considered in *Chapter 6*. This chapter looks at the duty of care in giving information to patients.

The duty of care to inform

The law of negligence is considered in *Chapter 4* where it is pointed out that a duty of care is owed to the patient. The duty of care includes not only a duty to treat, to diagnose, it also includes a duty to inform the patient of significant risks of substantial harm. Once a patient has given a valid consent to an operation proceeding, that consent would prevent an action for trespass to the person succeeding. However, if the patient has not been given information about the operation which would normally have been given by a health professional following the reasonable standard of care, then an action for negligence may succeed.

The claimant would have to prove on a balance of probabilities the following elements:

- a duty of care was owed to her to inform her of any significant risks of substantial harm
- there had been a breach of this duty in that the health professional had not given to her the information which any competent professional following the Bolam Test would have done
- as a consequence of this failure she agreed to have the operation, which she would not have done, had that information been given to her
- she has therefore suffered the harm of which she had not been warned.

Sidaway case

The leading case on the giving of information to a patient is that of *Sidaway* v. *Bethlem Royal Hospital Governors and others* [1985]. The facts are shown in *Box 10.2*.

Box 10.2: The facts of the Sidaway case

The claimant suffered chronic and intractable pain following an operation for a hernia repair. She was eventually referred to a specialist in pain relief who warned her of the possibility of disturbing a nerve root and the possible consequences of so doing but did not mention the possibility of damage to the spinal cord. The risk of spinal cord damage was less than 1%. She consented to the operation which was carried out by the surgeon with due care and skill. However, in the course of the operation she suffered injury to her spinal cord which resulted in her being severely disabled. She sued the surgeon for breach of his duty of care to warn her of all possible risks inherent in the operation.

The different judges in the House of Lords all had different bases for their views, but they agreed that in general she had failed in her action. Lord Diplock applied the Bolam principle to the duty of care to inform, Lord Bridge distinguished between two extremes: warning the patient of all possible risks and once the treatment has been decided upon in the patient's best interests, not warning the patient of any risks, in order not to alarm the patient. Between these two extremes, Lord Bridge suggested that the Bolam Test should be applied, but this did not mean handing over to the medical profession the entire question of the scope of the duty of disclosure. There will be circumstances where the judge could come to the conclusion that disclosure of a particular risk was so obviously necessary to an informed choice on the part of the patient that no reasonably prudent medical man would fail to make it. Lord Templeman stated that:

In my opinion, if a patient knows that a major operation may entail serious consequences, the patient cannot complain of lack of information unless the patient asks in vain for more information or unless there is some danger which by its

*nature or magnitude or for some other reason required to be
separately taken into account by the patient in order to reach
a balanced judgement in deciding whether or not to submit to
the operation.*

Lord Scarman supported a 'prudent patient test' a concept derived
from an American case, *Canterbury* v. *Spence*. In this case it was
recognised that there were four principles:

1. Every human being of adult years and of sound mind has a right
    to determine what shall be done with his own body.
2. The consent is the informed exercise of a choice and that entails
    an opportunity to evaluate knowledgeably the options available
    and the risks attendant on each.
3. The doctor must therefore disclose all 'material risks'; what
    risks are 'material' is determined by the 'prudent patient' test,
    which is as follows:

    A risk is... material when a reasonable person, in what the
    physician knows or should know to be the patient's position,
    would be likely to attach significance to the risk or cluster of
    risks in deciding whether or not to forgo the proposed therapy.

4. The doctor has, however, a therapeutic privilege. This exception
    is that a reasonable medical assessment of the patient would
    have indicated to the doctor that disclosure would have posed a
    serious threat of psychological detriment to the patient.

The House of Lords accepted that English law did not recognise the
doctrine of informed consent. Risks should be disclosed to enable the
patient to make a rational choice whether to undergo the particular
treatment recommended by a doctor. This duty was subject to the
doctor's overriding duty to have regard to the best interests of the
patient. Accordingly, it was for the doctor to decide what information
should be given to the patient and the terms in which that information
should be couched. The claimant therefore lost her appeal.

Application of the law to Mavis' situation

Mohammad signed the consent form knowing that an operation was to be carried out on his disc. He could not therefore succeed in an action for trespass to the person. Nor is it likely that he could succeed in an action for negligence for failures in the skill and care used in the operation, since he has no evidence that there were such failures. He may, however, succeed in an action for negligence alleging that there has been a breach of the duty of care to inform him of the significant risks of substantial harm which could occur from the disc operation. He would have to prove on a balance of probabilities that his surgeon failed to give him the information which any competent surgeon following the Bolam Test would have given. In addition, he would have to show that had he had that information and knew of the risk of harm, he would have refused to have had the operation.

Conclusion

The Kennedy Report of the paediatric heart surgery at Bristol Royal Infirmary emphasised that consent to treatment should be seen as a process and not simply the signing of a form. Feedback from patients should be encouraged. There should be a duty of candour, to tell a patient if adverse events have occurred and patients should receive an acknowledgement, an explanation and an apology. The implementation of such recommendations may move the legal position from the Bolam Test of giving information to the 'Prudent patient test' advocated by Lord Scarman in the Sidaway case.

Questions and exercises

❖ In what circumstances do you consider that information should be withheld from the patient?
❖ Do you follow any specific check list or principles when giving information to a patient about proposed treatment?
❖ Do you encourage patients to read the manufacturers' warnings about the medicines which you prescribe or administer?

References

Bristol Royal Infirmary Learning from Bristol; the report of the public inquiry into children's heart surgery at the Bristol Royal Infirmary 1984–1995 Command Paper CM 5207 July 2001; www.bristol-inquiry.org.uk/

Canterbury v. *Spence* 464 F 2d 772 (DC 1972)

Sidaway v. *Bethlem Royal Hospital Governors and others* [1985] 1 All ER 643

11

Letting die, killing and suicide

> ### Box 11.1: Case of *Re B.*
>
> Ms B. suffered a ruptured blood vessel in her neck which damaged her spinal cord. As a consequence she was paralysed from the neck down and was on a ventilator. She was of sound mind and knew that there was no cure for her condition. She asked for the ventilator to be switched off. Her doctors wished her to try out some special rehabilitation to improve the standard of her care and felt that an intensive care ward was not a suitable location for such a decision to be made. They were reluctant to perform such an action as switching off the ventilator without the court's approval. Ms B. applied for a declaration to be made that the ventilator could be switched off.

Introduction

In *Chapter 2* we considered the case of Diane Pretty who wanted her husband to be allowed to help her die. In this chapter we consider the law relating to murder and manslaughter and the legal distinction between letting die, killing, suicide and the right of autonomy of the mentally competent adult.

Murder

In order to secure a conviction of murder, the prosecution have to prove beyond all reasonable doubt that the defendant must either have intended to cause death or intended to cause grievous bodily harm. Unless a situation comparable to that of Dr Shipman, who was convicted of murdering fifteen patients, exists, it would be very unusual to be able to prove the intent necessary to convict of murder in a case involving professional care. Following a conviction for murder, a judge at the present time has no discretion over sentencing but must sentence the convicted person to life imprisonment, ie. a life sentence is mandatory.

Involuntary manslaughter

This may arise where death results from the gross negligence of a health professional, where there is no intention to kill or to cause grievous harm. In such cases there may be a prosecution for involuntary manslaughter or there may be no prosecution at all. It depends upon the circumstances. If, for example, there is such gross negligence leading to the death, then there may be a prosecution for manslaughter. The following two cases illustrate two different situations.

Death by misadventure

In 1991 two junior doctors were given a nine-month suspended prison sentence for the manslaughter of a sixteen-year-old with leukaemia. He died after being wrongly injected in the spine with a cytotoxic drug which should have been administered intra-venously. The conviction for manslaughter was quashed by the Court of Appeal on the ground that the jury should have been directed by the judge to decide whether the defendants were guilty of 'gross negligence' and not 'recklessness' and whether there were any mitigating circumstances, such as the lack of supervision from more experienced staff (*R. v. Prentice; R. v. Adomako; R. v. Holloway* [1993]).

Manslaughter

In the second case Dr Adomako, the person charged, was, during the latter part of an operation, the anaesthetist in charge of the patient. At approximately 11.05am a disconnection occurred at the endotracheal tube connection. The supply of oxygen to the patient ceased and led to a cardiac arrest at 11.14am. During that period the defendant failed to notice or remedy the disconnection. He first became aware that something was amiss when an alarm sounded on the Dinamap machine, which monitored the patient's blood pressure. From the evidence it appeared that some four and a half minutes would have elapsed between the disconnection and the sounding of the alarm. When the alarm sounded the defendant responded in various ways by checking the equipment and by administering atropine to raise the patient's pulse. But at no stage before the cardiac arrest did he check the integrity of the endotracheal tube connection. The disconnection was not discovered until after resuscitation measures had been commenced.

Dr Adomako accepted at his trial that he had been negligent. The issue was whether his conduct was criminal. He was convicted of involuntary manslaughter but appealed against his conviction. He lost his appeal in the Court of Appeal and then appealed to the House of Lords (*R. v. Adomako House of Lords* [1994]).

The House of Lords clarified the legal situation.

The stages which the House of Lords suggested should be followed were:

1. The ordinary principles of the law of negligence should be applied to ascertain whether or not the defendant had been in breach of a duty of care towards the victim who had died.

2. If such a breach of duty was established the next question was whether that breach of duty caused the death of the victim.
3. If so, the jury had to go on to consider whether that breach of duty should be characterised as gross negligence and therefore as a crime. That would depend on the seriousness of the breach of duty committed by the defendant in all the circumstances in which the defendant was placed when it occurred.
4. The jury would have to consider whether the extent to which the defendant's conduct departed from the proper standard of care incumbent upon him, involving as it must have done a risk of death to the patient, was such that it should be judged criminal.

The judge was required to give the jury a direction on the meaning of gross negligence as had been given in the present case by the Court of Appeal.

'The jury might properly find gross negligence on proof of:

a) indifference to an obvious risk of injury to health or of
b) actual foresight of the risk coupled either
      i. with a determination nevertheless to run it or
      ii. with an intention to avoid it but involving such a high degree of negligence in the attempted avoidance as the jury considered justified conviction or
c) of inattention or failure to advert to a serious risk going beyond mere inadvertence in respect of an obvious and important matter which the defendant's duty demanded he should address.'

(Lettering and numbering are the author's)

The House of Lords held that the Court of Appeal had applied the correct test and his appeal was dismissed.

The judge has full discretion over the sentencing in a case of conviction for involuntary manslaughter.

The case of Dr Nigel Cox

Dr Nigel Cox (*R. v. Cox* (1992)) was convicted when he prescribed and administered potassium chloride to a terminally ill patient and was sentenced to a year's imprisonment which was suspended for a year. He also had to appear before disciplinary proceedings of the Regional Health Authority, his employers and before the General Medical Council.

Voluntary manslaughter

This term is used to cover the situation where the defendant has caused the death of a person with intent, but owing to special circumstances a charge or conviction of murder is not appropriate. The term covers:

- death as a result of the provocation of the accused
- death as a result of diminished responsibility of the accused
- killing as a result of a suicide pact.

Letting die — the Tony Bland case

The House of Lords in the Tony Bland case (*Airedale NHS Trust* v. *Bland* [1993]) made it clear that there was in law a clear distinction between letting nature take its cause, when, in the light of the prognosis, it was in the best interests not to continue active interventions and killing the patient. In the word of Lord Goff:

> *The law draws a crucial distinction between cases in which a doctor decides not to provide, or to continue to provide, for*

his patient treatment or care which could or might prolong his life and those in which he decides, for example, by administering a lethal drug, actively to bring his patient's life to an end.

The facts of Tony Bland are shown in *Box 11.2.*

Box 11.2: Tony Bland

The patient was a victim of the football stadium crush at Hillsborough and it was established that although he could breathe and digest food independently, he could not see, hear, taste, smell or communicate in any way and it appeared that there was no hope of recovery or improvement. The House of Lords had to decide if it was lawful to permit artificial feeding to be discontinued in the case of a patient in a persistent vegetative state. The House of Lords decided that it would be in the best interests of the patient to discontinue the nasal gastric feed and he was later reported as having died.

A court in Bristol gave consent in a similar case a few months after the House of Lords decision in Tony Bland's case (*Frenchay Healthcare NHS Trust* v. *S.* [1994]).

Pain relief and killing

It does not follow that providing appropriate pain relief which may incidentally shorten life is a crime, as the trial of Dr Bodkin Adams made clear (*R.* v. *Adams Bodkin* [1957]). The facts are shown in *Box 11.3.*

> **Box 11.3: Dr Bodkin Adams**
>
> Dr Adams was charged with the murder of an elderly person receiving twenty-four-hour nursing care in Eastbourne. It was alleged that he gave her large quantities of morphia and heroin which caused her death.

In the case of Dr Bodkin Adams the trial judge Patrick Devlin directed the jury in the following words (Bedford, 1961):

If the first purpose of medicine — the restoration of health — can no longer be achieved, there is still much for the doctor to do, and he is entitled to do all that is proper and necessary to relieve pain and suffering even if the measures he takes may incidentally shorten life.... It remains a fact, and remains a law, that no doctor has the right to cut off life deliberately.... (the defence counsel) *was saying that the treatment given by the doctor was designed to promote comfort; and if it was the right and proper treatment of the case, the fact that incidentally it shortened life does not give any grounds for convicting him of murder.*

Dr Adams was found not guilty of murder.

Levels of medication

Clearly it must be established that the dosages which are given to a patient in the terminal stages of cancer and other illnesses are in accordance with the reasonable practice of a competent practitioner. It frequently happens that the tolerance built up to some pain medication requires higher and higher doses, which, given to persons without that tolerance would be lethal, grossly negligent and probably amount to a criminal offence. There is considerable benefit when practitioners are treating persons at such high levels to discuss recommended practice with colleagues. The importance of following competent medical practice is shown in the following case.

Annie Lindsell case

On 28 October 1997, Annie Lindsell (Wilkins, 1997) who was terminally ill with motor neurone disease applied to court for a declaration that her GP would not risk prosecution for murder if he gave her potentially lethal painkillers when her condition deteriorated. After hearing that a responsible body of medical opinion supported her GP's plan she withdrew her application for the court's intervention. In the case a clear distinction was made between pain relief whose principal purpose was to control her pain, even though incidentally it might shorten her life, and medication given to end her life. After the hearing, the British Medical Association (BMA) stated that it was pleased with the outcome, 'because it has confirmed that doctors working within the law, can treat the symptoms of terminally ill patients, even if that treatment may have a secondary consequence of shortening the patient's life.'

Annie Lindsell died a month later.

Suicide

As a result of the Suicide Act 1961, to attempt to commit suicide ceased to be a crime. However, the aiding and abetting of the suicide of another remained a criminal offence under section 2(1). This is shown in *Box 11.4*.

> **Box 11.4: Section 2(1) of the Suicide Act 1961**
>
> A person who aids, abets, counsels or procures the suicide of another, or an attempt by another to commit suicide, shall be liable on conviction of indictment to imprisonment for a term not exceeding fourteen years.

The patient's right of autonomy

In *Chapter 6* we consider the right of autonomy of the mentally capacitated patient and in *Chapter 9* the right of the mentally capacitated patient to refuse, by means of an advance direction, specified treatment if they subsequently lose their mental capacity. In the case of Diane Pretty which is discussed in *Chapter 2*, it is clear that she would have the right to refuse artificial feeding. However, she stated that she did not wish to suffer a slow death by starvation and would prefer to have a pain free, dignified and speedy death. In law she could lawfully attempt to commit suicide, but in practice she lacked the physical powers to do so. She needed to have assistance. Her application to the courts for a declaration that her husband should have an immunity from prosecution under section 2(1) of the Suicide Act 1969 were he to assist her to die, was refused. The House of Lords held that the Suicide Act was not contrary to her human rights as set out in the articles of the European Convention on Human Rights. She then applied unsuccessfully to the European Court of Human Rights in Strasbourg (*Chapter 2*).

Application of the law to the case in *Box 11.1*

It follows from this that Ms B., whose case is set out in *Box 11.1*, would have been able to refuse to go onto a ventilator. The anomalous situation which had arisen in her case was that she wished the ventilator to be switched off. She was mentally competent and was able to refuse treatment. Her doctors were reluctant to obey her instructions since it would appear that they would be aiding and abetting a suicide.

The High Court judge held that as a mentally competent adult she had a right to refuse even life-saving treatment. Ms B. was awarded a nominal sum of £100 for unlawful trespass. The ventilator could be switched off manually or mechanically and she would be given appropriate palliative drugs to permit her life to end peacefully and with dignity. Other hospitals had said that they would agree to do this. On 29 April 2002 it was announced that Ms B. had died peacefully in her sleep after the ventilator had been switched off (Bale, 2002).

The President of the Family Division, Dame Elizabeth Butler-Schloss, who heard the case of *Re B.*, restated the principles which had been laid down by the Court of Appeal in the case of St George's Healthcare Trust (*St George's Healthcare NHS Trust* v. *S.*):

- ❖ There was a presumption that a patient had the mental capacity to make decisions whether to consent to or refuse medical or surgical treatment offered.
- ❖ If mental capacity was not an issue and the patient, having been given the relevant information and offered the available option, chose to refuse that treatment, that decision had to be respected by the doctors; considerations of what the best interests of the patient would involve were irrelevant.
- ❖ Concern or doubts about the patient's mental capacity should be resolved as soon as possible by the doctors within the hospital or other normal medical procedures.

❖ Meanwhile the patient must be cared for in accordance with the judgement of the doctors as to the patient's best interests.

❖ It was most important that those considering the issue should not confuse the question of mental capacity with the nature of the decision made by the patient, however grave the consequences. Since the view of the patient might reflect a difference in values rather than an absence of competence, the assessment of capacity should be approached with that in mind and doctors should not allow an emotional reaction to, or strong disagreement with, the patient's decision to cloud their judgement in answering the primary question of capacity.

❖ Where disagreement still existed about competence, it was of the utmost importance that the patient be fully informed, involved and engaged in the process, which could involve obtaining independent outside help, of resolving the disagreement since the patient's involvement could be crucial to a good outcome.

❖ If the hospital was faced with a dilemma which doctors did not know how to resolve, that must be recognised and further steps taken as a matter of priority. Those in charge must not allow a situation of deadlock or drift to occur.

❖ If there was no disagreement about competence, but the doctors were for any reason unable to carry out the patient's wishes it was their duty to find other doctors who would do so.

❖ If all appropriate steps to seek independent assistance from medical experts outside the hospital had failed the hospital should not hesitate to make an application to the High Court or seek the advice of the Official Solicitor.

❖ The treating clinicians and the hospital should always have in mind that a seriously physically disabled patient who was mentally competent had the same right to personal autonomy and to make decisions as any other person with mental capacity.

Conclusion

To some philosophers in the ethics of health care, the present distinction in law between the legality of letting die (where appropriate) and the illegality of killing is not sustainable in logic, since death is the outcome of both, and killing may cause less suffering than letting nature take its course. The distinction is clearly apparent in a comparison of the cases of Diane Pretty and Ms B. The distinction is of extreme importance in the law and there is little likelihood of the law being changed in the near future.

Questions and exercises

❖ Do you consider that a competent adult could refuse every kind of care and treatment?

❖ What protection do you consider that the health professional and the patient should have when administering or receiving high dosages of medication?

❖ What are the advantages and disadvantages of introducing a law of euthanasia into this country?

References

Airedale NHS Trust v. *Bland* [1993] AC 789; [1993] 1 All ER 821

Bale J (2002) Miss B dies in peace after treatment ends. *The Times*, 30 April

Bedford S (1961) *The Best We Can Do*. Penguin, London

Frenchay Healthcare NHS Trust v. *S.* [1994] 2 All ER 403

Re B. (Consent to treatment: Capacity) The Times Law Report 26 March 2002

R. v. *Adams (Bodkin)* [1957] Crim LR 365

R. v. *Adomako House of Lords* The Times Law Report 4 July 1994; [1994] 2 All ER 79

R. v. *Cox (1992) 12 BMLR 38*

R. v. *Prentice*; *R.* v. *Adomako*; *R.* v. *Holloway* [1993] 4 All ER 935

St George's Healthcare NHS Trust v. *S.* The Times Law Report 8 May 1998, [1999] Fam 26

Wilkins E (1997) Dying woman granted wish for dignified end. *The Times*, 29 October

12

Confidentiality

Box 12.1: Situation

Jan was suffering from multiple sclerosis and in recent weeks had been suffering considerable pain and discomfort and her mobility was becoming increasingly impaired. She told her community nurse that she felt that she could not go on for much longer and was considering taking her own life. She did not ask the nurse for assistance, but requested that the nurse should keep this information confidential. What is the nurse's position in law.

Introduction

There are several sources which give rise to the duty of confidentiality which are recognised by all health professionals. They are explained in the author's book in this 'Legal Aspects of Health Care' series (Dimond, 2002). The duty of confidentiality derives from the trust which is created between patient and professional, from the professional codes of practice of registered health professionals and from specific statutory provisions. If there is a breach of confidentiality which is not justified in law, then the patient can apply for an injunction to prevent its publication, if in time; or, if not, sue for damages for the breach of confidentiality. In the case of *X.* v. *Y.* [1988], doctors working in the NHS who were suffering from AIDS were granted an injunction against a newspaper, preventing it publishing their names. The Court held that the information obtained from hospital records should be kept confidential and the public interest did not require the publication of the names. The Court did not order the disclosure by the press of their informant as the circumstances did not constitute one of the exceptional grounds on which the disclosure could be ordered against the press.

Exceptions to the duty of confidentiality

The basic presumption is that confidentiality should be respected but there are specific exceptions recognised both in statute and at common law. These include the following recognised exceptions:

- consent of the patient
- information given to other professionals in the interests of the patient
- order from the Court before or during legal proceedings
- statutory justification, eg:
    Notification of Registration of Births and Still Births
    Infectious Disease Regulations
    Police and Criminal Evidence Act
- public interest.

Consent of the patient

When the patient gives consent to the disclosure of confidential information, and the disclosure is made in accordance with this consent, then this would be a complete defence to any allegation of breach of confidentiality. There are clear advantages in obtaining the consent of the patient before disclosure is made.

Public interest

Even where the patient refuses to give consent to the disclosure, disclosure may be justified in the public interest. Where harm is feared to the patient or to another person, then the public interest would justify disclosure. For example, a concern that a child was at risk of being physically or mentally harmed would require disclosure to the appropriate child protection authorities. Most registration bodies of health practitioners recognise the 'public interest' as being a justification for the disclosure of confidential information. The Court of Appeal in the case of *W.* v. *Egdell* [1990] held that an independent psychiatrist who had sent his report to the Home Office and Medical Director of the hospital was justified in the public interest in making his findings known to those authorities.

Data Protection Act 1998

This Act applies to all patient records, both those held in manual format and those held on computer. All such records must comply with the data protection principles and the access provisions set out in statutory instruments (see below). The Information Commissioner combines the roles of Data Protection Commissioner enforcing the provisions of the Data Protection Act 1998, and Information Commissioner implementing the provisions (when brought into force) of the Freedom of Information Act 2000.

The Data Protection Act principles are shown in *Box 12.2*.

Box 12.2: Data Protection Act principles

1. Personal data shall be processed fairly and lawfully and, in particular, shall not be processed unless:
   a) at least one of the conditions in Schedule 2 is met; and
   b) in the case of sensitive personal data, at least one of the conditions in Schedule 3 is also met.
2. Personal data shall be obtained only for one or more specified and lawful purposes, and shall not be further processed in any manner incompatible with that purpose or those purposes.
3. Personal data shall be adequate, relevant and not excessive in relation to the purpose or purposes for which they are processed.
4. Personal data shall be accurate and, where necessary, kept up-to-date.
5. Personal data processed for any purpose or purposes shall not be kept for longer than is necessary for that purpose(s).
6. Personal data shall be processed in accordance with the rights of data subjects under this Act.
7. Appropriate technical and organisational measures shall be taken against unauthorised or unlawful processing of personal data and against accidental loss or destruction of, or damage to, personal data.
8. Personal data shall not be transferred to a country or territory outside the European Economic Area unless that country or territory ensures an adequate level of protection for the rights and freedom of data subjects in relation to the processing of personal data.

Access to personal health records

Section 7 of the Data Protection Act 1998 enables an individual to be informed of data held about him and to access that data. Special provisions exist in relation to health, education and social work under section 30. Section 30 enables the Secretary of State to draw up specific provisions setting exemptions from the statutory rights of access in relation to health, education and social work records. Statutory Instruments have been enacted setting out details of the restrictions on access to these records (Data Protection Orders, 2000).

Right to withhold access

Access can be withheld under the Data Protection Act 1998 in the following circumstances:

- where in the opinion of the holder of the record, serious harm would be caused to the mental or physical health or condition of the applicant or of any other individual
- where the identity of a third person would be made known and this person has not consented to access. (This does not apply where the other person is the health professional caring for the patient.)
- where the reports are confidential under a statutory provision, such as information supplied in a report or other evidence given to the court by a local authority, health or social services board, health and social services trust or probation officer.

Application of access provisions to a pain management situation

While there is a presumption in favour of access to health records, access could be refused if serious harm was feared. A patient who was terminally ill, but had not at that time been given the diagnosis, could be refused access if there was evidence that serious harm would be caused to his or her physical or mental health or condition. Such an exclusion from access would have to be justified in each case, since the patient has the right to challenge the refusal to provide access. A blanket policy of preventing access is legally invalid.

Application of the law to the situation in *Box 12.1*

Clearly, serious harm is feared to Jan if she continues with her suicide bid. The community nurse has a duty to ensure that Jan is receiving all the palliative care available. It may be that Jan needs to receive counselling assistance, since it may be that depression has undermined her mental capacity. She may benefit from further services for mobility and aid from the local authority. Jan has to use her professional discretion as to whether it is in Jan's interests for her suicide wishes to be made known to 'others' and who the appropriate 'others' may be. It may be that eventually Jan decides that her patient has all the care that she needs, and that her decision to take her own life is the result of clear thinking by a mentally competent person. If no other person is involved to assist (which would be a criminal offence) Jan may be justified in keeping the disclosure confidential. She may wish to seek advice and guidance from a senior manager or clinical supervisor. It is essential that she keeps clear, comprehensive records of her knowledge and her actions.

Conclusion

Whether a particular situation justifies a breach of confidentiality in the public interest is ultimately a question of professional discretion. Guidance is provided by the codes of practice and conduct issued by registration bodies, but the application of this guidance to a specific situation has to be decided by the individual practitioner who would be held personally and professionally accountable for his or her decision. Clear and comprehensive documentation is essential.

Questions and exercises

❖ In what circumstances would you breach the confidentiality of the patient? What would you tell the patient?
❖ Do you consider that there should be an absolute right of access for a patient to his or her health records?
❖ By 2005 the Government intends to introduce an individual patient electronic record. How would this affect your record keeping practice and what you record?

References

Data Protection (subject access modification) (health) Order 2000 SI 2000 No 413; Data Protection (subject access modification) (education) Order 2000 SI 2000 No 414; Data Protection (subject access modification (social work) Order 2000 SI 2000 No 415

Dimond B (2002) *Legal Aspects of Patient Confidentiality*. Quay Books, Mark Allen Publishing Limited, Salisbury, Wiltshire

W. v. *Egdell* [1990] 1 All ER 835

X. v. *Y*. [1988] 2 All ER 648

13

Medicines

Box 13.1: Situation

Augusta is a palliative care nurse who visits patients in the community advising them, their relatives and GPs on their care and arranging admissions to the hospice when appropriate. One patient is in the terminal stages of renal failure and on high doses of morphine. She is clearly in considerable discomfort and Augusta is asked by the patient if she could increase her dose. The patient does not wish her relatives to be told. Augusta is anxious to do this as soon as possible, since it may be several hours before the GP is able to visit. She phones the GP who tells her that she can give an additional dose and he would write it up later. Augusta administers this additional dose. Before the doctor has written up the additional dose, the patient dies. The relatives are now claiming that Augusta killed the patient. What is the law?

Introduction

The 1968 Medicines Act provided a statutory framework for the supply and control of medicines and sets out the classification of drugs. The Misuse of Drugs Act 1971 and subsequent legislation regulates the supply of specified controlled drugs. These statutes have been supplemented by Statutory Instruments providing more detailed regulation. The Medical Control Agency has the function of monitoring the safety and quality of medicines. Its website provides access for health professionals, members of the public, academics, the pharmaceutical industry and journalists (www.open.gov.uk/mca/mcahome.htm). It operates a Defective Medicines Report Centre.

While initially under the Medicines Act 1968 the only recognised professions for prescribing medications were doctors, dentists, veterinary surgeons and midwives, recent legislation has expanded approved prescribers.

Nurse prescribing

Following the first Crown Report (Report on Nurse Prescribing and Supply, 1989) the powers of prescribing were extended to nurses and health visitors. The Medicinal Products (Nurse Prescribing etc) Act 1992 enables a registered nurse, either health visitor or district nurse, who has the requisite additional training to prescribe those medicinal products contained in a nurse's formulary, set out in a Schedule to the Prescription Only Medicines Order (Statutory Instrument, 1994). Section 58 of the Medicines Act 1968 (as amended by the 1992 Act) enables an appropriate practitioner to provide a prescription to be dispensed by the registered pharmacist. Nurse prescribing in the community has a clear statutory basis and can take place within certain clearly defined parameters (Dimond, 1995). In February 2000, an amendment by Statutory Instrument added nurses employed by a doctor whose name is included in a medical list (eg. practice nurses) and those assisting in the capacity of a nurse, in the provision of services in a walk-in centre (defined as a centre at which information and treatment for minor conditions is provided to the public under arrangements made by or on behalf of the Secretary of State) to the group of nurses who were recognised as being able to prescribe after the appropriate training had been given.

Second Crown Report and patient group directions

Dr Crown was appointed in 1997 to chair a committee to review prescribing, supply and administration of medicines. Its terms of reference included the development of a consistent policy framework to guide judgements on the circumstances in which health professionals might undertake new responsibilities with regard to prescribing, supply and administration of medicines. It was also asked to advise on the likely impact of any proposed changes; to consider possible implications for legislation, professional training and standards and to advise on prescription etc under group protocols and on any safeguards.

Its initial report was published in 1998 and was concerned with the prescribing, supply and administration under group protocols (DoH, 1998). It recommended that the majority of patients should continue to receive medicines on an individual basis. However, current safe and effective practice using group protocols which are consistent with criteria defined in the Report should continue. As a consequence of this interim Report, a statutory instrument was published specifying the minimum requirements for a patient group direction (originally known as group protocol). These requirements are shown in *Box 13.2*.

One developing role of the practitioner specialising in pain management is the transcribing of patient group directions on ward drug charts for nurse prescribing. The specialist nurse could, within the agreed patient group direction, amend the drug charts to suit the changing needs of the patient and write up drugs for ward charts to be administered by the ward nurses.

Box 13.2: Particulars for Patient Group Direction

a. The period during which the Direction shall have effect
b. The description or class of prescription only medicines to which the Direction relates
c. Whether there are any restrictions on the quantity of medicine which may be supplied on any one occasion, and if so, what restrictions
d. The clinical situations which prescription only medicines of that description or class may be used to treat
e. The clinical criteria under which a person shall be eligible for treatment
f. Whether any class of person is excluded from treatment under the Direction, and if so, what class of person
g. Whether there are circumstances in which further advice should be sought from a doctor or dentist and, if so, what circumstances
h. The pharmaceutical form or forms in which prescription only medicines of that description or class are to be administered
i. The strength, or maximum strength, at which prescription only medicines of that description or class are to be administered
j. The applicable dosage or maximum dosage
k. The route of administration
l. The frequency of administration
m. Any minimum or maximum period of administration applicable to prescription only medicines of that description or class
n. Whether there are any relevant warnings to note, and if so, what warnings
o. Whether there is any follow-up action to be taken in any circumstances, and if so, what action and in what circumstances
p. Arrangements for referral for medical advice
q. Details of the records to be kept of the supply or the administration of medicines under the Direction.

The Final Crown Report

The recommendations of the Final Report of the Crown Committee (DoH, 1999) included the following recommendations:

1. The legal authority in the UK to prescribe should be extended beyond currently authorised prescribers.
2. The legal authority to prescribe should be limited to medicines in specific therapeutic areas related to particular competence and expertise of the group.
3. Two types of prescribers should be recognised: the independent prescriber and the dependent prescriber.
4. A UK-wide advisory body, provisionally entitled the 'New Prescribers Advisory Committee' should be established under section 4 of the Medicines Act to assess submissions from professional organisations seeking powers for suitably trained members to become independent or dependent prescribers.
5. Newly authorised groups of prescribers should not normally be allowed to prescribe specified categories of medicines including controlled drugs.
6. The current arrangements for the administration and self-administration of medicines should continue to apply. Newly authorised prescribers should have the power to administer those parenteral prescription only medicines which they are authorised to prescribe.

As a consequence of these recommendations, legislation is contained in section 63 of the Health and Social Care Act which amends the Medicines Act 1968. It amends section 58 of the Medicines Act to enable 'other persons who are of such a description and comply with such conditions as may be specified in the order' to be eligible to write prescriptions for medicinal products.

Section 63(3) lists those persons who are eligible as including persons who are registered by a board established under the Professions

Supplementary to Medicine Act 1960 or by a body set up under the Health Act 1999 (for example, the HPC or NMC).

Extended formulary nurse prescribers

Further developments in extending prescribing powers came into force on 1 April 2002. A statutory instrument laid down arrangements for a nurse registered in Parts 1, 3, 5, 8, 10, 11, 12, 13, 14, or 15 of the professional register and who is recorded in the register as qualified to order drugs, medicines and appliances from the extended formulary to prescribe products listed in the extended formulary. Schedule 3A of the statutory instrument sets out the substances which may be prescribed, administered or directed for administration by extended formulary nurse prescibers. The Schedule also sets out the conditions for such prescription or administration. The list includes antibiotics, analgesics and vaccines. Full details are published in the *BNF*. In brief, the extended formulary nurse prescribers are able to prescribe all pharmacy and general sales list medicines prescribable by a GP and also those prescription only medicines (PoMs) which are set out in Schedule 3A of the Order. These cover minor injuries, minor ailments, health promotion and palliative care.

Guidance on extending independent nurse prescribing within the NHS in England

Guidance was issued in March 2002 by the Department of Health (DoH, 2002). It covers such topics as:

- who may prescribe and what
- implementation strategy
- education and training
- action for employers

- prescription form
- security and handling of prescription forms
- good practice
- nursing records
- adverse reaction reporting
- legal and clinical liability
- dispensing of prescribed items
- verification of prescribing status
- dispensing and budget setting and monitoring.

It is highly likely that many palliative care practitioners will, after the appropriate training which is financed from central funds, be eligible to become extended formulary nurse prescribers. Fuller details of the Department of Health guidance is available from its website.

Future developments

On 16 April 2002 the Department of Health published proposals to give nurses and pharmacists further prescribing powers to cover some chronic conditions. The proposals are to be implemented in 2003 and will enable appropriately trained nurses and pharmacists to prescribe for such conditions as asthma, diabetes, high blood pressure and arthritis. Prescriptions for inhalers, hormone replacement therapy and anti-coagulants are included in the proposals. Public consultation on the proposals is due to end in July 2002.

Application of the law to the situation of Augusta

At present, even if Augusta had powers of prescribing in the community the nurse's formulary does not include controlled drugs. It may be that eventually as the extended formulary and supplementary prescribing powers are further extended then independent nurse prescribers will have the powers to vary the dose of controlled drugs given by the GP or to decide the dose in her own right. At the present time Augusta is clearly guilty of misconduct. She should have waited for the doctor to attend the patient. It is, however, unlikely that her actions caused the death of the patient (although this would have to be investigated). She would face disciplinary actions before her employers and also professional conduct proceedings before the NMC.

Conclusion

Significant extensions of prescribing powers are now in place under the Extended Formulary Nurse Prescribing rules. At the time of writing further supplementary prescribing powers are under consultation. There are dangers in too rapid an extension of prescribing powers leading to harm to patients. It is essential that there should be sufficient training and that prescribers should always work within their competence and ensure that they keep up-to-date on information about the substances they can prescribe. It is likely that these developments will have a major impact upon the role of the palliative care nurse and all those health professionals concerned with pain management.

Questions and exercises

- ❖ To what extent do you consider that your powers to prescribe could be extended or initiated?
- ❖ Do you consider the present provisions for the safety of medicines provide adequate protection for the patient?
- ❖ How much information do you give a patient about the potential side-effects of medication? (refer also to *Chapter 10*).

References

Department of Health (1989) *Report on Nurse Prescribing and Supply*. Advisory group chaired by Dr June Crown. DoH, London

Department of Health (1998) *Review of Prescribing, Supplying and Administration of Medicines. A Report on the Supply and Administration of Medicines under Group Protocols*. Chaired by Dr June Crown. DoH, London: April

Department of Health (1999) *Review of Prescribing, Supply and Administration of Medicines. Final report*. Chaired by Dr June Crown. DoH, London: March

Department of Health (2002) *Extending Independent Nurse Prescribing within the NHS in England: a guide for implementation*. DoH, London: March

Department of Health guidance on nurse prescribers online at: www.doh.gov.uk/nurseprescribing/implementationguide.htm

Dimond B (1995) *Nurse Prescribing*. Merck Dermatology and Scutari Press, London

Statutory Instrument 1994 No 3050 The Medicines (Products other than Veterinary Drugs) (Prescription Only) Amendment (No 3) Order 1994. HMSO, London

Statutory Instrument 2000 No 121 The National Health Service (Pharmaceutical Services) Amendment Regulations 2000. HMSO, London

Statutory Instrument 2002 No 549 The Prescription Only Medicines (Human Use) Amendment Order 2002. The Stationery Office, London

14

Complementary therapies

Box 14.1: Situation

Noel was a pain control nurse who with his colleagues provided a specialist service to the district hospital, being brought in by the wards and departments to assist in advising on pain management. In addition to his nursing qualifications, he had also studied acupuncture and was able to offer an acupuncture service to the patients. Following one course of treatment, a patient complained that a needle had caused paralysis to her arm and she stated that she would sue for compensation. What is the legal position of Noel?

Introduction

The popularity and growth in use of complementary and alternative therapies over recent years is a remarkable phenomenon. An information pack for primary care on complementary medicine has been sponsored by the Department of Health (2000). The pack was initiated after a survey found that one in four adults would use alternative therapies at some point in their lives. The Health Education Authority (HEA) has published an A to Z guide which covers sixty therapies (HEA, 1995).

The House of Lords select committee on science and technology held an inquiry into complementary medicine. It reported in November 2000 and recommended that there should be regulations of complementary and alternative medicines (CAM) and there should be further research to evaluate their effectiveness. It divided such therapies into three groups:

❖ Professionally organised therapies, where there is some scientific evidence of their success, though seldom of the highest quality and there are recognised systems for treatment and training of practitioners. This group includes acupuncture, chiropractic herbal medicine, homeopathy and osteopathy.
❖ Complementary medicines, where evidence that they work is generally lacking but which are used as an adjunct rather than a replacement for conventional therapies, so that lack of evidence may not matter so much. Included in this group are; Alexander Technique, aromatherapy, nutritional medicine, hypnotherapy and Bach and other flower remedies.
❖ Techniques that offer diagnosis as well as treatment, but for which scientific evidence is almost completely lacking. This group cannot be supported and includes; naturopathy, crystal therapy, kinesiology, radionics, dowsing and iridology.

The Select Committee of the House of Lords considered that some remedies such as acupuncture and aromatherapy should be available on the NHS and NHS patients should have wider access to osteopathy and chiropractics.

The British Medical Association at its conference in 2000 also recommended that acupuncture should be available on the NHS.

Two aspects of complementary and alternative therapy use

The practitioner in pain management needs to be aware of two separate issues which may arise in the use of complementary therapies. One is the legal implications if she herself becomes a practitioner of such therapies as Noel in *Box 14.1*. The other is the legal significance of a patient utilising complementary therapies in addition to the orthodox treatments provided under the NHS. This latter situation shall be considered first.

Patients using complementary therapies

Practitioners in pain management (referred to as pain practitioners) may discover quite by chance that their patients are also trying out various complementary or alternative therapies. There are possible dangers because certain orthodox treatments may be contraindicated if the patient is receiving other treatments. For example, if a physiotherapist is assisting a patient who has chronic back pain, there may be conflicts with treatment provided by a chiropractic practitioner. It is advisable for the pain practitioner to obtain the patient's consent to contact the other practitioner in order to ensure that there are no conflicts between the different treatment plans. Should the patient refuse to give such consent, or refuse to allow records to be exchanged between the two practitioners, then the pain practitioner might have to advise the patient that because of potential dangers, she could not continue to treat the patient in ignorance of the plan being followed by the other practitioner.

It is essential that the pain practitioner is aware of the significance of the other treatments being given to the patient and acquires as much knowledge as possible about them.

The pain practitioner as complementary therapist

Where the pain practitioner develops skills in a complementary therapy and wishes to practise this as part of her NHS work, it is essential that the employer is aware of her intentions and gives approval. Without this approval, should harm result from negligent practice of the complementary therapy, the employer may be able to argue that this therapy was practised outside the course of employment and it is therefore not vicariously liable for it (*Chapter 4*). Many NHS Trusts now have a procedure for checking on the competence of an employee to practise a specific complementary therapy as part of his or her employment and for giving approval to that. It is preferable to obtain such approval in writing. Sometimes the NHS trust may insist that the patient specifically gives consent to this treatment. For example, an NHS trust may insist that all patients give consent before a complementary therapy is used upon them. A nurse who is skilled in aromatherapy, might consider that her skills could bring comfort to patients in the intensive care unit. However, it is unlikely that consent could be obtained before the patient is placed on the ventilator, and therefore she would be unable to provide aromatherapy for such patients. At the present time, until such therapies become part of orthodox medicine, it would not be possible to argue that they are in the best interests of a mentally incapacitated patient and could be given to unconscious patients without their consent.

Application of the law to the situation of Noel in *Box 14.1*

Noel will have to establish that his work as an acupuncturist was carried out with the knowledge and the express or implied consent of the employer. If he can establish this he can argue that he was acting in the course of his employment in providing the acupuncture services. If it can be shown that the patient's paralysis was a reasonably foreseeable result of negligence on his part, then his employer would be vicariously liable for his negligence and would have to pay compensation to the patient. (It may of course be that the paralysis was not caused by the acupuncture needle, in which case the claimant would not succeed in an action for compensation [*Chapter 4*].) On the other hand, if Noel is unable to show that he was acting in the course of employment (this would be particularly so, if he took payment from the patients and was acting as a self-employed practitioner in this work), then he is personally accountable for the harm which has been caused and would have to rely upon his own indemnity insurance cover. If he lacked such insurance cover, then his home and other possessions could be put at risk.

Conclusion

The implementation of the recommendations of the Select Committee of the House of Lords will lead to fundamental changes in how complementary and alternative therapies are viewed in relation to orthodox medicine and within the NHS. It is essential that pain practitioners who wish to practice in these fields are sure of their competence to do so and take steps to obtain the written agreement of their employer to use these therapies in addition to the skills from their registered professions.

Questions and exercises

❖ Establish whether your employer has a check list and procedure to ensure the competence and approval for those employees who wish to practice complementary or alternative therapies.
❖ How do you prove that you are competent in a complementary or alternative therapy?
❖ Which complementary and alternative therapies, if any, do you consider should be available on the NHS and why?

References

Department of Health (2000) *Complementary medicine: information pack for primary care groups.* DoH, London; www.doh.gov.uk

Health Education Authority (1995) *A–Z Guide on Complementary Therapies.* HEA, London

House of Lords Select Committee on Science and Technology 6th Report Complementary and Alternative Medicine 21 November 2000 Session 1999–2000

15

Scope of professional practice

Box 15.1: Situation

Marcus is a registered physiotherapist specialising in musculo-skeletal problems. He would find it useful to prescribe a sedative to his patients before he treats them. At present he has to arrange for the patient to be written up for such medication by the doctor. He is seeking prescribing powers. What is the law?

Introduction

It is likely that as the developments envisaged in *The NHS Plan* (Secretary of State for Health, 2000) take effect, the significance of the original training of a registered practitioner count for less than the post registration training and experience. Many healthcare activities may be undertaken by practitioners from a variety of registered professions. The Government's plans for the NHS as shown in the White Paper (DoH, 1997), in the document *Making a Difference* (DoH, 1999) and in *The NHS Plan* rely heavily upon a widened scope of practice for the nurse and other health professions. NHS Direct and walk-in clinics are run by nurses and provide an increasingly extensive and popular service. Standards and organisational issues are considered in *Chapter 17*.

Statutory provisions

Unless an Act of Parliament or other statutory provision requires an activity to be undertaken by a specific health professional, then, provided the necessary training, experience and knowledge are acquired so that the activity could be undertaken competently, any registered health professional could undertake that activity. There are very few statutes which require activities to be performed only by a practitioner of a specified registered profession. One of these is the Mental Health Act 1983. Under section 5(2) of this Act only the registered medical practitioner treating the patient or a registered medical practitioner nominated by the former can detain an informal patient for up to seventy-two hours. Similar provisions specify that it must be a registered medical practitioner providing the medical recommendations for detaining a patient and determining treatment under Part IV of the Act. The Abortion Act 1967 requires an approved termination to be carried out by a registered medical practitioner, but the House of Lords (*Royal College of Nursing* v. *Department of Health and Social Security* [1981]) interpreted this as meaning that the doctor responsible for the termination when prostaglandins were being administered could supervise its being carried out by a nurse. As Lord Diplock said in the House of Lords:

> *The doctor need not do everything with his own hands; the subsection's requirements were satisfied when the treatment was one prescribed by a registered medical practitioner carried out in accordance with his directions and of which he remained in charge throughout.*

The Medicines Act 1968, as we saw in *Chapter 13*, is also specific as to which named professions could undertake activities under the Act, but section 63 of the Health and Social Care Act 2001 has extended the provisions of section 58 of the Medicines Act 1968 to enable other registered health practitioners to have prescribing powers. At the time of writing the publication of the regulations, which will specify the conditions under which these practitioners can prescribe, is awaited.

Prescribing powers

The extension of prescribing powers to additional professions will have a major impact upon role definition. Already, those practitioners identified in the statutory instrument relating to patient group directions can prescribe against an agreed protocol. These new regulations came into force on 9 August 2000. Regulations clarifying independent and dependent prescribers and the conditions of their prescribing are implemented then pain practitioners may find their roles are considerably enhanced (*Chapter 13*).

Other areas of role expansion

Other areas in which the pain practitioner may develop her skills include:

- triage of patients in A&E
- nurse led pain relief clinics, for example, in acupuncture, transcutaneous electric nerve stimulation (TENS)
- spinal cord implant clinics
- transcribing from group protocols on to the ward drug charts (*Chapter 13*)
- audit on records for pain assessment and management (*Chapter 19*).

Conditions for developing the scope of professional practice

Where an activity is undertaken by a different professional than the one who would normally undertake that activity, the law requires that the same standard of the competent professional as per the Bolam Test is followed. It is no defence to argue that a person with less training or experience carried out that activity, if harm to the patient occurs. The patient is entitled to expect that he or she would receive the reasonable standard of care whoever is undertaking that activity. The UKCC laid down principles for the safe development of the scope of professional practice, which are relevant to all healthcare professionals (*Box 15.2*). These principles are now incorporated in the *Code of professional conduct* of the NMC (2002).

Application of the law to the situation in *Box 15.1*

Marcus may be able to agree with the doctors treating his patients, that a patient group direction should be drawn up in accordance with the requirements as shown in *Box 13.2 (p. 87)*, which would enable him to give appropriate medication before treating his patients. He would need to follow the principles laid down in *Box 15.2* to ensure that he is competent to undertake this activity safely. Ultimately, it may be that he could be identified as an independent or dependent practitioner in his particular field of work and be recognised as having wider prescribing powers.

Conclusion

In its report 'Anaesthesia under Examination', the Audit Commission made significant recommendations on anaesthetic and pain management services and suggested that there was considerable scope for the role expansion of many of the different professional groups who work in theatres. The Audit Commission Report illustrates how problems can arise when inter-disciplinary team-working breaks down. It puts forward practical suggestions on how trusts can improve anaesthetic and pain relief services.

Box 15.2: Principles for adjusting the *Scope of Professional Practice*

The registered nurse, midwife or health visitor:

1. must be satisfied that each aspect of practice is directed to meeting the needs and serving the interests of the patient or client;
2. must endeavour always to achieve, maintain and develop knowledge, skill and competence to respond to those needs and interests;
3. must honestly acknowledge any limits of personal knowledge and skill and take steps to remedy any relevant deficits in order effectively and appropriately to meet the needs of patients and clients;
4. must ensure that any enlargement or adjustment of the scope of personal professional practice must be achieved without compromising or fragmenting existing aspects of professional practice and care and that requirements of the Council's *Code of professional conduct* are satisfied throughout the whole area of practice;
5. must recognise and honour the direct or indirect personal accountability borne for all aspects of professional practice, and;
6. must serve the interests of patients and clients and the wider interests of society, avoid any inappropriate delegation to others which compromises those interests.

The competence of the individual practitioner caring for the patient provides the protection of the patient. That practitioner must work within his or her field of competence, acknowledging any gaps in knowledge and expertise and ensure that the necessary additional training, supervised practice and experience are obtained. Major developments can be expected in the next few years and it is essential that there is on-going multidisciplinary discussions to ensure co-ordination of who is doing what, and when, in patient care and particularly pain management.

Questions and exercises

❖ In what ways do you consider that the scope of your professional practice could be developed?
❖ How would you determine your competence to undertake any specific expanded role activity?
❖ How can professionals ensure that there is co-ordination when several different professionals are able to undertake the same activities?

References

Audit Commission (1997) *Anaesthesia under Examination: The efficiency and effectiveness of anaesthesia and pain relief services in England and Wales.* Audit Commission, London: 17 December

Department of Health (1997) *The New NHS — modern, dependable.* DoH, London

Department of Health (1999) *Making a Difference. Strengthening the nursing, midwifery and health visiting contribution to health and health care.* DoH, London

Royal College of Nursing of the UK v. *Department of Health and Social Security* [1981] AC 800; [1981] 1 All ER 545

Secretary of State for Health (2000) The NHS Plan Cm 4818-1. The Stationery Office, London: July

Statutory Instrument 2000 No 1917 Prescription only Medicines (Human Use) Amendment Order. HMSO, London

Health and safety and consumer protection

Introduction

Health and safety laws which protect the health and safety of employees, patients and the general public derive from many statutory and common law sources but the principle legislation is the Health and Safety at Work Act 1974 (HASWA) and statutory instruments made under it. Section 2 places a duty on the employer to take reasonable care of the health safety and welfare of its employees, and section 3 places a duty on the employer to all those whose health or safety may be affected by its enterprise. Under section 7 each employee has a duty to take reasonable care of the health and safety of himself and others and to co-operate with the employer in obeying health and safety laws. These statutory duties are enforced by way of criminal proceedings by the Health and Safety Executive and its inspectors. These statutory duties are paralleled by duties under the contract of employment under which the employer has an implied duty to take reasonable care for the health and safety of the employee and the employee a duty to obey the reasonable instructions of the employer; and by the laws of negligence, where a duty of care is owed to patients and others (as we have seen in *Chapter 4*) . Other statutory provisions cover the liability of the occupier to visitors (Occupier's Liability Act 1957) and to trespassers (Occupier's Liability Act 1984), the regulations relating to substances hazardous to health, the reporting of incidents of disease and the medical devices regulations. These are considered in more detail in the author's law books for nurses, midwives, physiotherapists and occupational therapists (see *Further reading*).

Relevance of health and safety laws to pain practitioners

Health and safety laws are relevant to pain practitioners whatever their registered profession. They need to have an understanding of the laws which apply to them and from whom they can obtain further information. For example, many pain practitioners may be involved in manual handling; assisting a patient into a more comfortable position may not be lifting, but would come within the definition of manual handling. The pain practitioner needs to have an understanding of how such an action can be undertaken safely and the basic legal requirements of the manual handling regulations. One example of statutory provision taken to indicate the relevance of these laws to pain practitioners is the Management of Health and Safety in the Workplace Regulations 1999.

Management of Health and Safety in the Workplace Regulations 1999

These regulations require each employer to undertake a suitable and sufficient assessment of the risks to the health and safety of his employees. Suitable and sufficient are not defined within the regulations, but the *Approved Code of Practice and Guidance* gives practical advice on how to carry out a risk assessment (Health and Safety Commission [HSC], 1999, 2000).

Medical devices regulations

Almost all the equipment used by pain practitioners would come within the definition of a medical device. The definition used by the Medical Devices Agency (MDA) is based upon the European Directive definition (European Union Directive 93/42/EC):

Any instrument, apparatus, material or other article, whether used alone or in combination, including the software necessary for its proper application, intended by the manufacturer to be used for human beings for the purpose of:

- diagnosis, prevention, monitoring, treatment or alleviation of disease
- diagnosis, monitoring, treatment, alleviation of or compensation for an injury or handicap
- investigation, replacement or modification of the anatomy or of a physiological process
- control of contraception.

and which does not achieve its principal intended action in or on the human body by pharmacological, immunological or metabolic means, but which may be assisted in its function by such means.

The pain practitioner must ensure that she is aware of any warning notices which are issued by the Medical Devices Agency. She must also ensure that she is aware of the procedure for the notification of any defects and who is her liaison officer for the purposes of the MDA regulations.

National Patient Safety Agency (NPSA)

The NPSA was established in 2001 to run the mandatory reporting system for logging all failures, mistakes, errors and near misses across the health services (DoH, 2001a). The Department of Health's publication *Building a Safer NHS for Patients* (DoH, 2001b) sets out details of the scheme together with recommendations for an improved system for handling investigations and inquiries across the NHS. Eventually it will incorporate the statutory reports required under health and safety legislation. The aim is to ensure that the NHS learns from all adverse incidents which occur across the country.

Consumer Protection Act 1987

The Consumer Protection Act 1987 enables a claim to be brought where harm has occurred as a result of a defect in a product. It is a form of strict liability in that negligence by the supplier or manufacture does not have to be established. The claimant will, however, have to show that there was a defect. The supplier can rely upon a defence colloquially known as 'state of the art', ie. that the state of scientific and technical knowledge at the time the goods were supplied was not such that the producer of products of that kind might be expected to have discovered the defect. The claim is brought against the manufacturer or supplier of the goods. A successful claim was brought in March 1993 (Dimond, 1993) when Simon Garratt was awarded £1,400 against the manufacturers of a pair of surgical scissors which broke during an operation on his knee, with the blade being left embedded. A second operation was required to remove it. Had he relied upon the law of negligence to obtain compensation he would have had to show that the manufacturers were in breach of the duty of care which they owed to him.

More recently, patients who had contracted hepatitis C from blood and blood products used in blood transfusions brought a case (*A. and others* v. *National Blood Authority and another*) under the Consumer Protection Act 1987 and succeeded. This decision may well lead to greater use of the Consumer Protection Act 1987 where personal injuries are caused as a result of defective products. Negligence does not have to be established under the Consumer Protection Act 1987, only that there was a defect in the product which has caused the harm.

Application of the law to the situation in *Box 16.1*

The patient has many possible causes of action in this situation. There may well be a possible claim in negligence against the employer of Serena who is vicariously liable for the negligence of Serena. It would have to be shown that Serena was in breach of the duty of care which she owed to the patient. There may be considerable difficulties in establishing that Serena was in breach of the duty of care. Alternatively and probably more effectively, the patient could bring an action against the suppliers or manufacturers of the needles. She would need to be given details of the product from the hospital: the name and address of the manufacturers or suppliers and if possible the batch numbers. If the hospital is unable to provide this information, then it becomes the supplier for the purposes of the Consumer Protection Act 1987. Serena must ensure that notification of the defect is made to the hospital liaison officer who is in contact with the Medical Devices Agency. In addition, a report should be made to the National Patient Safety Agency.

Conclusions

It will be evident that this chapter has barely touched the surface of the vast body of legislation and case law which applies to health and safety and the practitioner is referred to relevant works cited on *page 145*. Regular contact with the NHS trust health and safety officer would ensure that the practitioner keeps up-to-date.

Questions and exercises

❖ Check the record of accidents which have taken place over the past month and consider the extent to which these could have been avoided.

❖ Observe your practice for a week and the types of equipment and instruments which would come within the definition of a medical device. Ensure that you regularly receive notifications from the MDA.

❖ How do the Management of Health and Safety Regulations apply to your work?

References

A. and others v. *National Blood Authority and another* The Times Law Report 4 April 2001

Department of Health (2001a) Press release. *National patient safety agency to be launched*. DoH, London

Department of Health (2001b) *Building a Safer NHS for Patients*. DoH, London

Dimond B (1993) Protecting the consumer. *Nurs Standard* **7**(24): 18–19

Health and Safety Commission (1999) Management of Health and Safety at Work Regulations 1999. HSC, London

Health and Safety Commission (2000) *Approved Code of Practice and Guidance 2000*. HSC, London

17

Standards and organisational issues

Box 17.1: Situation

Mustafa suffered considerable pain while he was in hospital and was appalled to discover that there was no pain management service provided by the hospital. He understood that the trust board was under a statutory duty to lay down and monitor standards of quality and was considering suing the board for its failure to provide a reasonable service and fulfil its statutory obligations.

Introduction

In *Chapter 15* we considered developments in the scope of professional practice in the light of Government plans as shown in the White Paper (DoH, 1997), and in the documents *Making a Difference.* (DoH, 1999) and *The NHS Plan* (DoH, 2000). Legislation implementing these plans is to be found in the Health Act 1999, the Health and Social Care Act 2001 and the NHS Reform and Health Care Profession Bill 2002. Over recent years the following have been initiated: the National Institute for Clinical Excellence, the Commission for Health Improvement, the National Service Frameworks, the National Patient Safety Agency and many others.

Clinical governance

One of the most important initiatives was the introduction of the concept of clinical governance. It derives from the statutory duty under section 18 of the Health Act 1999 (*Box 17.2*).

> **Box 17.2: Section 18 Health Act 1999**
>
> It is the duty of each health authority, primary care trust and NHS trust to put and keep in place arrangements for the purpose of monitoring and improving the quality of health care which it provides to individuals.

The duty falls primarily upon the chief executive of each health authority and NHS trust.

The result of this statutory duty is that NHS trust boards and their chief officers are responsible for the standard of clinical care within the organisation. If they fail to ensure that reasonable standards of care are in place, then the board and its chairman and chief officers can be replaced by the Secretary of State. As a consequence of this power greater freedom has been granted to those NHS Trusts whose hospitals have reached high standards in the league tables and the management of poor performers (DoH, 2002a) has been taken over. In 2002 the zero rated trusts were given three months to show clear signs of improvement. Those which failed to show such improvements had their management taken over by successful managers from other trusts or from the private sector (DoH, 2002b).

National Institute of Clinical Excellence (NICE)

This organisation was established on 1 April 1999 to promote clinical and cost effectiveness. The then Secretary of State stated that its task would be to abolish postcode variation in the country, so that there would be national standards for the provision of health care such as medicines. One of the functions of NICE is to issue clinical guidelines and clinical audit methodologies and information on good practice. The National Institute for Clinical Excellence has a major role to play in the setting of standards of practice, by disseminating the results of research of what is proved to be clinically effective, research-based practice. It is essential that pain practitioners are aware of the reports and recommendations of NICE. It does not follow that they will automatically become binding on practitioners, since practitioners will still have to use their professional discretion in deciding whether the guidelines are appropriate for the care and treatment of the individual patient. However, if the practitioner fails to follow the guidelines, she would have to give clear reasons why they were not appropriate for the circumstances of that individual patient. It is likely that as its work progresses, more of its recommendations whether on medications or clinical procedures will relate to pain management. Claimants may be able to show that there has been a breach of the duty of care which has caused harm by establishing that NICE guidelines were ignored.

Commission for Health Improvement (CHI)

Sections 19 to 24 of the Health Act 1999 establish the Commission for Health Improvement and sets out its functions and powers. It is a body corporate, ie. it can sue and be sued on its own account. It undertakes inspections of NHS trusts, health authorities and primary care trusts over a five-year cycle and will carry out additional inspections at the request of the Secretary of State. Its reports are likely to influence standards of health care provision across the NHS. It was asked by the Department of Health in 2001 to inspect policies on 'Not For Resuscitation' when it made its inspection visits to NHS trusts.

National Service Frameworks (NSF)

NSFs have been set up for several specialties including; mental health, coronary heart disease, cancer care and older peoples' services. NSFs for diabetes and for maternity and child health are under preparation. Pain management may eventually have its own NSF or be included in several different NSFs. The NSF sets minimum standards to be achieved across the specific specialty and could become a major justification for the redistribution of resources. For example in pain management, if pain practitioners were aware that an NSF recommended that in each hospital there should be a central service for pain management advice and treatment, then this could be used as justification for the allocation of resources for such a service.

Kennedy Report

The report on paediatric heart surgery in Bristol (Bristol Royal Infirmary, 2001) has made significant recommendations for a fundamental change in the relationship between patients and professionals within the NHS. Implementation of these recommendations should ensure that there is openness and honesty between professional and patient and where concerns are raised these are dealt with honestly. Patients should be told of untoward events.

Application of the law to the situation in *Box 17.1*

Mustafa may well have an action in negligence if he can show that there was a failure to follow the reasonable standard of care in controlling his pain. If he can establish that the ward staff did not follow basic principles of pain management and as a consequence he suffered additional harm, then he may have grounds for suing the trust for its vicarious liability for the negligence of its staff. He may also have an action for breach of the direct liability of the trust to him for its failure to establish a safe system for pain management in its hospital. This latter cause of action would be more problematic in its success. It is unlikely that the courts would see that an individual patient had a right to sue a trust for breach of its statutory duty under section 18 of the Health Act 1999. Usually, breach of a statutory duty is not open as a cause of action to a claimant if there are other remedies. In this statute other remedies would include the right of the Secretary of State to remove the trust board, or for the claimant to pursue a complaint against the trust. The handling of complaints is considered in the next chapter.

Conclusion

The significant changes which have taken place in the NHS over the last few years have placed considerable pressures upon practitioners to be aware of recommendations, advice guidelines, procedures and protocols issued by the new institutions. Ignorance of recommended practice would be no defence to a practitioner if such advice had become incorporated into the standards of the reasonable practitioner as set out in the Bolam Test.

Questions and exercises

❖ Examine the extent to which NICE recommendations relate to pain management.

❖ A CHI inspection is due to take place in your trust over the next three months. What preparations would you make for such a visit and how would it help you ensure a high standard of care for your patients?

❖ To what extent has the NSF for the care of cancer patients been implemented in your trust and how has it effected your practice?

References

Bristol Royal Infirmary (2001) Learning from Bristol: the report of the public inquiry into children's heart surgery at the Bristol Royal Infirmary 1984–1995. Command paper CM 5207, July 2001; www.bristol-inquiry.org.uk/

Department of Health (1997) *The New NHS — modern, dependable*. DoH, London

Department of Health (1999) *Making a Difference. Strengthening the nursing, midwifery and health visiting contribution to health and healthcare*. DoH, London

Department of Health (2002a) Press release. *Milburn announces radical decentralisation of NHS control*. DoH, London

Department of Health (2002b) Press release 0069. DoH, London

Secretary of State for Health (2000) The NHS Plan Cm 4818-1. The Stationery Office, London: July

18

Complaints and patient representation

> **Box 18.1: Situation**
>
> Sunny was admitted to hospital for the birth of her first child, though she had hoped to have had a home birth. Subsequently, she complained that she had been given an epidural without her consent and had wanted to have minimum intervention. She asked the midwife for her complaint to be investigated.

Introduction

The Hospital Complaints Act 1985 sought to ensure that in each hospital there was an effective procedure for dealing with complaints by patients and their representatives and was followed by guidance recommending that the complaints machinery should also be extended to community health services. In 1994 the recommendations of the Wilson Committee (DoH, 1994) for dealing with hospital and primary care complaints were implemented in the establishment in 1996 of a complaints procedure. Subsequently, in the National Plan the Government stated that it was to establish a National Patient Safety Agency to set up a full mandatory reporting scheme for adverse healthcare events (*Chapter 17*), improved professional regulatory mechanisms for doctors and other health professionals (*Chapter 5*), and a new patient advocacy service.

Chapter 10 of *The NHS Plan* sets out the strategy for implementing significant changes for patient care. These include:

- more information for patients

- greater patient choice
- patients' advocates and advisers in every hospital
- redress over cancelled operations
- patients' forums and citizens' panels in every trust
- new national panel to advise on major reorganisations of hospitals.
- stronger regulation of professional standards.

These changes, some of which need legislative provision, are slowly being implemented.

Patient Information Advisory Group

One of the first innovations to take place is the establishment of a Patient Information Advisory Group (Statutory Instrument 2001 No 2836) under regulations drawn up by the Secretary of State under powers given by sections 61 and 64 of the Health and Social Care Act 2001. The Advisory Group will consist of not less than twelve or more than twenty members and will meet at least four times a year. Its principal function is to give advice to the Secretary of State on draft regulations drawn up under section 60 of the Health and Social Care Act 2001. These regulations enable the Secretary of State to control the processing of prescribed patient information for medical purposes as he considers necessary in the interests of improving patient care or in the public interest.

Patient Advocacy and Liaison Services (PALS)

Another significant proposal is the Patient Advocacy and Liaison Services (PALS). *The NHS Plan* envisages that by 2002 PALS will be established in every major hospital with an annual national budget of around £10 million. A new patient advocacy team, usually situated in the main reception areas of hospitals, will act as a welcoming point for patients and carers and a clearly identifiable information point. Patient advocates will act as an independent facilitator to handle patient and family concerns, with direct access to the chief executive and the power to negotiate immediate solutions. They will work with other organisation such as the Citizens Advice Bureau.

Patients' forums

These are to be set up in every NHS trust and primary care trust to provide direct input from patients about how local NHS services are run. Patients will have direct representation on every NHS trust board. The representatives will be elected by the patients' forum. The forum will be supported by each PALS and will have the right to visit and inspect any aspect of the trust's care at any time.

Community Health Councils

It was originally intended that PALS would replace the Community Health Councils (although the National Assembly for Wales is not taking this route). A consultation paper, 'Involving patients and the public in healthcare' (DoH, 2001a) was issued by the Department of Health in September 2001 for consultation on proposals for greater public representation to replace the CHCs. In a press release on 3 September 2001 (DoH, 2001b), the Department of Health announced that a new independent body 'Voice' was to be established. There would be two levels:

❖ At national level a new national body called Voice — the Commission for Patient and Public Involvement in Health.
❖ At local level there will be local bodies called Voice which will report patients' concerns from PALS and forums to the new strategic health authorities.

Voice will set national standards and monitor local services, helping to ensure communities have an effective say in their local NHS. Voice will work alongside the trust based patients' forums and patient advocacy and liaison services. The NHS Reform and Healthcare Professions Bill makes provision for the abolition of Community Health Councils in England. Clearly, these changes will have to fit in with plans to reform the current patients' complaints system.

Complaints procedure

Several years ago research was commissioned by the Department of Health on the effectiveness of the current complaints system. In the light of the results of that research the Department of Health published a document suggesting a number of ways to improve the current procedure (DoH, 2001c). It also issued a consultation document on which feedback was invited. It is likely to lead to significant changes to the present complaints system in 2002.

Application of the law to the situation in *Box 18.1*

It is advisable for Sunny to be asked to put her complaint in writing, but even if it is just a complaint by word of mouth it should be properly investigated. Under the present scheme for handling complaints, there would be an attempt to resolve it at a local level.

There would be a thorough investigation in which the midwife would be asked for a detailed account of what happened, the condition of Sunny and her requests. Following this investigation the results would be reported to Sunny. If Sunny were not satisfied with the response she would have the right to ask the non-executive director of the trust who was the convenor of complaints to consider whether an independent review panel (IRP) could be established. If this request was refused or if Sunny were not satisfied with the outcome from the IRP she would be able to take her complaint to the Health Service Commissioner, known as the Ombudsman. There may be significant changes to this procedure following the recent review carried out by the Department of Health. Sunny may find that she has a right of legal redress because of her complaint, since the investigation may reveal that she has an action for trespass to her person and/or an action for negligence in her care which has caused her harm. If this is revealed during the complaints process, Sunny may well have to decide whether to pursue the complaints process or initiate litigation instead.

Conclusion

Major changes are taking place in patient representation with the establishment of new patient organisations. These are likely to have a significant effect on the way in which complaints are handled. Pain practitioners who are confident in their practice will welcome improved communication between patients and professionals and the establishment of these new organisations.

Questions and exercises

❖ Examine complaints received over the past month. To what extent can lessons be learnt from these complaints and improvements put in hand?
❖ What benefits do you consider a patient's representative could bring to the service which you provide?
❖ How could you obtain effective feedback on the service which you give to the patients?

References

Department of Health (1994) *Being Heard*. The report of a review committee chaired by Professor Wilson on NHS complaints procedures. DoH, London

Department of Health (2001a) *Involving Patients and the Public in Healthcare*. DoH, London: 3 September

Department of Health (2001b) Press release. *New Voice for Patients to Shape Local Services*. DoH, London: 3 September

Department of Health (2001c) *NHS Complaints Procedure — National Evaluation*. DoH, London

Department of Health (2001d) *Reforming the NHS Complaints Procedure: A Listening Document*. DoH, London

Secretary of State for Health (2000) The NHS Plan Cm 4818-1. The Stationery Office, London: July

Statutory Instrument 2001 No 2836 Patient Information Advisory Group (Establishment) Regulations 2001

19

Record keeping

Introduction

There are few statutory provisions which apply to standards and the nature of documentation in health care. Exceptions include regulations under the Mental Health Act 1983 which requires statutory documents to be kept for detention and consent to treatment, and under the Abortion Act 1967 which also specifies which particulars are statutorily required. Apart from such exceptions, the law relating to standards of record keeping derives from the common law concerning the reasonable standard of professional practice and guidance issued by registration bodies and professional associations.

Basic principles

The basic principle on which standards of record keeping rest is the care of the patient. The UKCC (1998) emphasised that good record keeping helps to protect the welfare of patients and clients by promoting:

- high standards of clinical care
- continuity of care
- better communication and dissemination of information between members of the inter-professional healthcare team
- an accurate account of treatment and care planning and delivery
- the ability to detect problems, such as changes in the patient's or client's condition, at an early stage.

Guidance is provided by the UKCC (*Box 19.2*) and is relevant to all healthcare practitioners, not just nurses, midwives and health visitors.

Guidance is also provided in the former NHS Training Directorate booklets (NHS Training Directorate, 1995) and by the NHS Executive. The Audit Commission made recommendations to improve the standard of record keeping in hospitals in 1995 (Audit Commission, 1995). It reviewed the situation in 1999 and concluded that although progress had been made there was still scope for further improvements (Audit Commission, 1999).

The Clinical Negligence Scheme for Trusts inspects the record keeping standards of those trusts who are members of the scheme and provides helpful guidance on standards.

Box 19.2: UKCC principles for record keeping (1998)

Patient and client records should:

- ❖ Be factual, consistent and accurate.
- ❖ Be written as soon as possible after an event has occurred, providing current information on the care and condition of the patient or client.
- ❖ Be written clearly and in such a manner that the text cannot be erased.
- ❖ Be written in such a manner that any alterations or additions are dated, timed and signed in such a way that the original entry can still be read clearly.
- ❖ Be accurately dated, timed and signed, with the signature printed alongside the first entry.
- ❖ Not include abbreviations, jargon, meaningless phrases, irrelevant speculation and offensive subjective statements.
- ❖ Be readable on any photocopies.

In addition, records should:

- ❖ Be written, wherever possible, with the involvement of the patient or client or their carer.
- ❖ Be written in terms that the patient or client can understand.
- ❖ Be consecutive.
- ❖ Identify problems that have arisen and the action taken to rectify them.
- ❖ Provide clear evidence of the the care planned, the decisions made, the care delivered and the information shared.

Monitoring standards

Regular internal audit on record keeping standards is a useful method of identifying and maintaining standards. Internal audit can be supported by external reviews by the King's Fund, other management consultancy organisations and the Commission for Health Improvement (*Chapter 17*). To be effective the audit should be repeated at frequent intervals to identify if suggested changes are being implemented and standards improved.

Prescribing

There are many decided cases where harm has been caused to a patient as a result of handwriting which has been misread by a pharmacist. For example, in one case (*Prendergast* v. *Sam & Dee Ltd* [1989]) the doctor prescribed amoxil (an antibiotic) for the patient which, because of bad handwriting, was misread as daonil (a drug used by diabetics) by the pharmacist. As a consequence of the wrong medication the patient suffered from severe hypoglycaemia and brain damage from oxygen shortage in the blood. The doctor was held 25% to blame and the pharmacist 75%. The latter should have been alerted to the misreading because of the dosage and the fact that the patient paid for the prescription. £119,302 was paid out in compensation. In another case (Kennedy, 1996) a junior doctor and staff nurse misread the dose written up for a patient who had had a hysterectomy. The consultant had prescribed a top up epidural of 3mgs of diamorphine in 10mls of saline, the junior doctor misread this as 30mgs. The patient died.

As more and more practitioners extend their professional roles to include prescribing powers, good handwriting will become essential. Eventually computer records and computer-generated prescriptions may avoid the necessity for reliance on hand-written prescriptions and documentation.

A prescription

Advice is given in the *British National Formulary* (*BNF*) on the writing of prescriptions:

'Prescriptions should be

- written legibly in ink or otherwise so as to be indelible
- should be dated
- should state the full name and address of the patient
- should be signed in ink by the prescriber
- the age and the date of birth of the patient should preferably be stated and it is a legal requirement in the case of prescription-only medicine to state the age for children under twelve years.'

The *BNF* also gives advice on the writing of dosages, the use of abbreviations and on computer-issued prescriptions. It notes that computer-generated facsimile signatures do not meet legal requirements.

Records used in pain management

Information about the pain suffered by the patient should be included in the following records:

- general observations of the patient's condition (often kept at the bed side)
- nursing and medical records setting out treatment plans, prescription charts and pain scores and management
- audit records by pain practitioners often using pro formas or hand held computers
- specific records for patients on patient controlled analgesia
- specific records for epidural analgesia and patients with special problems.

The pain practitioner can have a valuable role in standard setting and monitoring by carrying out regular audit with ward colleagues on the completion of records and the recording of pain levels and its management.

Application of the law to the situation in *Box 19.1*

It is apparent that the failure to record levels of pain suffered by the patient is a major defect in the record keeping standards of those caring for Marius. If there had been appropriate recording, it may have been that the failure to calibrate the syringe driver at the correct level would have come to light much earlier in the patient's treatment. The complaint would appear to be soundly based and the trust should ensure that an apology is given. It should also give an assurance that staff training will be undertaken to prevent such a mistake reoccurring.

Conclusion

Good standards of record keeping are part of the practitioner's professional duty of care to the patient. If a good standard is maintained in the clarity and comprehensiveness of the entries, then it is likely that, if there is a complaint, or litigation or other hearing, the documentation would provide adequate evidence for use before these hearings so as to explain the conduct and actions of the practitioner. However, like health and safety practice, there has to be constant monitoring to ensure that standards do not fall.

Questions and exercises

❖ Examine the extent to which you and your colleagues' record keeping satisfies the standards of reasonable practice.
❖ What differences would it make to your record keeping practice, if all patients were responsible for the safeguarding of their records?
❖ How frequently is an audit carried out of record keeping standards in your department? Could it be made more effective?

References

Audit Commission (1995) *Setting the Records Straight: A study of hospital medical records*. Audit Commission, Abingdon

Audit Commission (1999) *Update Setting the Records Straight*. Audit Commission, Abingdon

British Medical Association and Royal Pharmaceutical Society of Great Britain *British National Formulary*. Updated and published annually. BMA, London

Health and Safety Commission 1998/217 *Preservation, Retention and Destruction of GP Medical Services Records Relating to Patients*

Health and Safety Commission 1999/053 *For the Record: Managing records in NHS Trusts and Health Authorities*

NHS Training Directorate (1995) *Just for the Record*. NHS Training Division

Kennedy D (1996) Hospital blamed in report on overdose death. *The Times*, 3 July

Prendergast v. *Sam & Dee Ltd* [1989] 1 Med LR 36

United Kingdom Central Council for Nursing, Midwifery and Health Visiting (1998) *Guidelines for Records and Record Keeping*. UKCC, London, reprinted by NMC, 2002

20

Research

Box 20.1: Situation

Ortis was employed as a pharmacist in a district general hospital. She was aware that a drug trial was taking place in the hospital on a new analgesic. She was dispensing this to a patient and asked the patient if she was aware that the drug was part of a research project. The patient stated that she had no knowledge of any such research but was taking the medicine for her arthritis. What should Ortis do?

Introduction

Research into both medication and treatment regimes is likely to become more and more a feature of patient care. Reasonable standards of care require that where possible research-based clinically effective practice is followed, which necessitates increasing random control testing for many procedures whose efficacy is assumed rather than established through clear research. As a consequence, many pain practitioners might find that they themselves are involved in a research project, or if not, they are caring for patients who are the research subjects in a colleague's research project.

All the principles of law which have been considered in this book, apply to the patient who is asked to participate in a research project. Of particular concern is the law relating to consent, confidentiality and liability if harm to the patient should occur. See

Further reading (p. 145) for detailed discussion on these and other legal issues. As part of the clinical governance initiative, the Department of Health has published a research governance framework (DoH, 2001). This sets out the responsibilities of a research sponsor and requires that organisations willing to take on these duties to be included on a list of recognised sponsors complete a base line assessment. The framework seeks to establish standards for all those involved in research in health and social care.

Law relating to research

The Human Rights Act 1998 (*Chapter 2*) and all other statutes and common law decisions also apply to the rights of data subjects. In addition, there are statutory regulations for the carrying out of research on animals (Animals (Scientific Procedures) Act 1986) and for the testing of medicinal products (Medicines Act 1968), and for testing on embryos (Human Fertilisation and Embryology Act 1990).

Declarations and guidance

Many declarations from international conventions and guidelines from professional registration bodies or associations also cover research practice. These declarations and guidelines, while they are frequently incorporated into the standards of professional practice, are not in themselves directly enforceable in the courts in this country. For example, two of the principle conventions covering the practice of research are the Nuremberg Code and the Declaration of Helsinki. Ten principles, which should be observed in order to satisfy moral, ethical and legal concepts, were laid down by the Nuremberg Courts following the military trials which took place at the end of the Second

World War. These principles have become known as the Nuremberg Code (Kennedy and Grubb, 2000) and are summarised in *Box 20.2*.

Box 20.2: Principles for research from Nuremberg Code

1. The voluntary consent of the human subject is absolutely essential.
2. The experiment should be such as to yield fruitful results for the good of society, unprocurable by other methods.
3. The experiment should be based on results of animal experiments and a knowledge of the natural history of the disease or other problem so that the anticipated results should justify the performance of the experiment.
4. The experiment should be so conducted as to avoid all unnecessary physical and mental suffering and injury.
5. No experiment should be conducted where there is an *a priori* reason to believe that death or disabling injury will occur; except, perhaps, in those circumstances where the experimental physicians also serve as subjects.
6. The degree of risk to be taken should never exceed that determined by the humanitarian importance of the problem to be solved by the experiment.
7. Proper preparations should be made and adequate facilities provided to protect the experimental subject against even remote possibilities of injury, disability or death.
8. The experiment should be conducted only by a scientifically qualified person. The highest degree of skill and care should be required through all stages of the experiment of those who conduct or engage in the experiment.
9. During the course of the experiment the human subject should be at liberty to bring the experiment to an end if he had reached the physical or mental state where continuation of the experiment seems to him to be impossible.
10. During the course of the experiment the scientist in charge must be prepared to terminate the experiment at any stage, if he has probable cause to believe, in the exercise of good faith, superior skill and careful judgement required of him that a continuation of the experiment is likely to result in injury, disability, or death to the experimental subject.

Subsequently, the World Medical Association published a Declaration of Helsinki in 1964 which set out principles for the carrying out of research on human subjects. Amendments were made in 2000 following a conference in Edinburgh (European Forum for Good Clinical Practice, 1999). While the Declaration of Helsinki is not directly binding on the courts of this country (as the European Convention on Human Rights is through the Human Rights Act 1998), local ethics committees and researchers would have regard to its principles when giving agreement to and embarking on a research project.

Most health professional registration bodies and professional associations have drawn up guidelines for undertaking research. For example, the Standards Committee of the GMC has drafted guidance on medical research: the role and responsibilities of doctors, which is obtainable from the GMC website.

Consent

All those principles relating to the consent of the patient and the giving of information to the patient prior to any project starting (considered in *Chapters 6–10*) apply. Special provisions relate to any research on children and unless there are clear therapeutic benefits to a child, it is doubtful if a parent has the right in law to give consent on behalf of their children to research which may carry risks where these are not offset by therapeutic benefits. The United Nations Convention on the Rights of the Child was drawn up in 1989 (United Nations Convention, 1989) and ratified by the UK in 1991. It represents clear guidance for the development of rights-based and child-centred health care.

There are advantages in a researcher obtaining the services of an independent person to explain the project and obtain a valid consent.

Confidentiality

Information obtained from the patient during the research project is subject to exactly the same laws on confidentiality as are discussed in *Chapter 12*. The same exceptions to the duty apply and justification for disclosure in the public interest would exist if serious harm to the patient or to other persons were feared.

Liability for harm

Even though the Pearson Report in 1978 recommended that both volunteers and patients who take part in medical research and clinical trials and who suffer severe damage as a result should receive compensation on the basis of strict liability, this recommendation has never been implemented in law. Most research initiated by pharmaceutical companies is, however, conducted on the basis that compensation would be paid to those who were harmed as a result of participation in a research project without the research subject having to prove fault and the local research ethics committee (LREC) would ensure that this agreement was signed.

Local research ethics committees

The Department of Health has requested that each health authority ensure that an LREC (DoH, 1991) is set up to examine research proposals. All those involved in research projects whether as actual researchers or as carers for patients who are research subjects should ensure that there has been LREC approval to the project. Some research is conducted on a multi-centred basis and multi-centre research ethics committees (MRECs), established by the Department of Health, oversee research which is carried on across several LREC catchment areas. Where less than five LRECs are involved, one LREC can act on behalf of the others.

Application of the law to the situation in *Box 20.1*

It is clear that there are real concerns to Ortis as to whether the patient has been given sufficient information about the medicines she is taking and the fact that she is participating in a research project. Ortis should raise these concerns with the doctor. It may well be that the research is being carried out on a multi-centred basis. However, that is no justification for failing to ensure that each patient has been given the relevant information about the project and has given a valid consent. With support from her manager, Ortis could make it clear that the pharmacy department will not dispense medications to patients which are being used on a trial basis, unless the patients have clearly been told about the research and have had an opportunity to consent to or refuse participation in the research.

Conclusion

There is a considerable range of guidance both international, national and professional on undertaking research. It may be that in future more of this guidance will be brought into legislation and become legally binding upon researchers and more easily enforceable by the patient. The new patient organisations considered in *Chapter 17* are also likely to become involved in ensuring that research projects recognise and protect the rights of the patient. The openness and integrity called for by the Kennedy Report into the paediatric heart surgery at Bristol should be at the heart of any research project.

Questions and exercises

❖ How do you ensure that your practice keeps pace with accepted research findings?

❖ If you were caring for a patient who was taking part in a research project what action would you take to ensure that the rights of the patient were protected?

❖ You have been asked to assist in a research project. What issues would you clarify before you commenced your work?

References

Bristol Royal Infirmary (2001) Learning from Bristol: the report of the public inquiry into children's heart surgery at the Bristol Royal Infirmary 1984–1995. Command paper CM 5207, July 2001; www.bristol-inquiry.org.uk/

Department of Health (1991) Local Research Ethics Committees HSG(91)5. DoH, London

Department of Health (2001) Research Governance Framework. DoH, London; www.doh.gov.uk/research/rd3/nhsrandd/researchgovernance.htm

European Forum for Good Clinical Practice Bulletin of Medical Ethics Revising the Declaration of Helsinki: a fresh start. London: 3–4 September, 1999

Kennedy I, Grubb A (2000) *Medical Law*. 3rd edn. Butterworths, London

Royal Commission on Civil Liability and Compensation for Personal Injury Chaired by Lord Pearson Cmnd 7054 1978 HMSO, London

United Nations Convention on the Rights of the Child 20. Xi 1989; TS 44; Cm 1976

21

Social security and other financial provisions

Box 21.1: Situation

Jim knows that he is likely to die very soon and wants to ensure that his relatives are not financially burdened by his care during his final weeks. He therefore wishes to find out the benefits to which he is entitled to ensure an application is made for these as soon as possible.

Introduction

There are a bewildering array of benefits available from your health authority (for example, travelling expenses to hospital) from the Department for Work and Pensions (in which there is a business unit known as the Disability and Carers Directorate), the local authority, the Department of Trade and Industry and the Inland Revenue (tax credits). Each benefit has its own conditions of entitlement, some are backdated, some only payable from the date a claim has been made. Any person who gives advice in this area must ensure that it is up-to-date. It is preferable to give individuals the source of where advice can be obtained rather than pretend to have full comprehensive up-to-date knowledge.

The following information is only a brief outline of the benefits currently available and further details should be obtained from the relevant departments.

Benefits fall into one of three categories:

1. Benefits available as of right.
2. Benefits available on a means tested basis, either through social security or the local authority.
3. Benefits which are work related and eligibility depends upon meeting certain criteria relating to length of continuous service and other conditions laid down in the legislation.

Benefits available to all

Disability Living Allowance (DLA)

This is available on a non-means tested basis for persons who are under sixty-five years and who need help with personal care or getting around because they are ill or disabled. The care component is paid at three levels and the mobility component at two levels. Special Rules enable a person to receive highest rate care without delay and without enduring a qualifying benefit. This is payable to a person who has a terminal illness and is not expected to live for more than six months. A special DS1500 medical report completed by a doctor must be submitted. A mobility payment may also be made.

Attendance Allowance (AA)

This is available for disabled people aged sixty-five and over who need help with personal care because of their illness or disability. Normally the help must have been needed for at least six months. The special provision (see under 'DLA') for those with a terminal illness is also available under the Attendance Allowance.

Incapacity Benefit

This is available to those who are ineligible for the statutory sick pay scheme.

Benefits which are means tested

Income support

This is available to people on a low income, who are over sixteen years and not working (or working less than sixteen hours a week).

Lone parent run-on

An extra two weeks payment for lone parents who stop getting income support or income-based job-seekers allowance because they start to work or increase their working for sixteen hours a week or more.

Working families and Disabled persons tax credit

Payable through the inland revenue as a deduction for tax payable in respect of working people who are bringing up children or to people who have a long-term health problem.

The Social Fund

There are two elements to the fund:

The Regulated Social Fund

Grants are available to those who satisfy the rules of entitlement. They include payments for maternity expenses, funeral expenses, periods of cold weather and winter fuel.

The Discretionary Social Fund

Payments can be in the form of grants or interest free loans. Community care grants are available to those on income support to assist in coming out of institutional care or to avoid going into an institution.

Budgeting loans are interest free loans to assist in one-off purchases, such as beds and cookers. Crisis loans are available to those faced with an emergency or crisis. Unlike budgeting loans, crisis loans are available to those who are not on income support as well as those who are.

Invalidity care allowance

This is available for persons between sixteen and sixty-five who are spending at least thirty-five hours a week caring for a severely disabled person who is in receipt of the middle or highest level of DLA care component or AA.

Council tax benefit

Local authorities will reduce the amount payable in council tax for those who are on low incomes or who live on their own. Disabled people and carers may also receive discounts on council tax.

Housing benefit

This is paid by the local council for people who need help with rent. The amount payable depends upon the means of the claimant and the general level of rents in the area for that type of property.

Health benefits

The following are available to specified groups or those on low incomes receiving income support:

- free prescriptions
- free NHS dental treatment
- free NHS sight test
- voucher towards cost of glasses or contact lenses
- free NHS wigs and fabric supports
- travel costs to and from hospital.

Benefits which are work related

In addition, there are benefits such as maternity payments and leave and statutory sick pay which are available for employees.

Collection of benefits

Arrangements can be made for another person to collect benefit by nominating an appointee to be recognised by the local post office. Alternatively, an official Power of Attorney can be submitted or the claimant can name another person whom they would like to receive their benefit on their behalf. A person can authorise the collection of the benefit from the post office by signing the book of the order or the claimant can request direct payment to their bank account.

Application of the law to *Box 21.1*

Urgent advice should be obtained for Jim on the benefits which are available to him. If he is under sixty-five he may be eligible for a disability living allowance and the special provision for those who are terminally ill. If he is over sixty-five then the attendance allowance may be available as well as the allowance for the terminally ill.

Requests for application packs should be made as soon as possible to the appropriate Disability Benefits centre, benefits agency (a section of the Department of Work and Pensions) or local council.

Charitable grants

In addition to the help already mentioned there are charities and trusts who will consider giving financial help to a patient and his/her family. Such help is normally means tested and can cover a wide variety of practicable needs. Social workers or welfare rights officers should be able to provide information on their availability.

Conclusion

Pain practitioners will find it useful to know who can be contacted to provide detailed advice to their patients. Social workers who specialise in benefits or welfare rights officers should be able to provide up-to-date expertise on the way through the benefits maze. Other sources of advice would be; the Disability Benefit Helpline on 0800 882200, local Social Security offices, (see local telephone directory under Benefit agency, Social Security office or Department of Work and Pensions) or Citizens Advice Bureau. At a time when a patient is gravely ill and facing death, it is essential that they do not have to cope with financial worries and uncertainties: knowledgeable, speedy assistance is vital to the patient and his or her family.

Questions and exercises

❖ Find out where you can obtain up-to-date advice on benefits for patients receiving palliative care.

❖ How can the interests of the patient be protected when relatives are obtaining the benefits on the patient's behalf? (You may need to seek the advice of the Benefits Agency on this.)

❖ What are the legal consequences if you give misleading advice to a patient which results in their losing some benefits to which they would have been entitled had they applied in time? (See *Chapters 4* and *10*.)

Conclusions

This succinct book does not pretend to cover in detail all aspects of the law relating to pain management. The intention has been to introduce the law to those who are not familiar with its jargon and its content and to provide a ready reference to others who need to refresh their knowledge. It is hoped that practitioners will be able to follow this book up by referring to some of the more detailed works contained in the list of *Further reading*. Inevitably, new statutes are passed, new cases decided and the law moves on. It is imperative, as in other aspects of their professional practice, that the practitioner keeps up-to-date with these changes. If this book has opened up a subject which is seen by many as forbidding and threatening and if it has enabled practitioners to pursue their work of pain management with greater confidence in using the law to protect their patients, their colleagues and themselves, then it will have served its purpose.

Bridgit Dimond
May, 2002

Further reading

Brazier M (1992) *Medicine, Patients and the Law*. Penguin, London

Card R, Cross, Jones (1998) *Criminal Law*. 14th edn. Butterworths, London

Denis IH (1999) *The Law of Evidence*. Sweet and Maxwell London

Dimond BC (1999) *Patients' Rights, Responsibilities and the Nurse*. 2nd edn. Quay Books, Mark Allen Publishing Ltd, Salisbury, Wiltshire

Dimond BC (1997) *Legal Aspects of Occupational Therapy*. Blackwell Science, Oxford

Dimond BC (1996) *Legal Aspects of Child Health Care*. Mosby, London

Dimond BC (2002) *Legal Aspects of Midwifery*. 2nd edn. Books for Midwives Press/Butterworth Heinemann, Oxford

Dimond BC, Barker F (1996) *Mental Health Law for Nurses*. Blackwell Science, Oxford

Dimond BC (1997) *Legal Aspects of Care in the Community*. Macmillan Publishers, London

Dimond BC (1998) *Legal Aspects of Complementary Therapy Practice*. Churchill Livingstone, Edinburgh

Dimond BC (2002) *Legal Aspects of Nursing*. Pearson Education, London

Dimond BC (1999) *Legal Aspects of Physiotherapy*. Blackwell Science, Oxford

Finch J (ed) (1994) *Speller's Law Relating to Hospitals*. 7th edn. Chapman and Hall Medical, London

Harris P (1997) *An Introduction to Law*. 5th edn. Butterworths, London

Hunt G, Wainwright P (eds) (1994) *Expanding the Role of the Nurse*. Blackwell Science, Oxford

Hurwitz B (1998) *Clinical Guidelines and the Law*. Radcliffe Medical Press, Oxford

Ingman T (1996) *The English Legal Process*. 6th edn. Blackstone Publishing, London

Jones R (12001) *Mental Health Law Manual*. 7th edn. Sweet and Maxwell, London

Kennedy I, Grubb A (2000) *Medical Law and Ethics*. 3rd edn. Butterworths, London

Kennedy T (1998) *Learning European Law*. Sweet and Maxwell, London

Kloss D (2000) *Occupational Health Law*. 3rd edn. Blackwell Science, Oxford

Knight B (1992) *Legal Aspects of Medical Practice*. 5th edn. Churchill Livingstone, Edinburgh

Markesinis BS, Deakin SF (1999) *Tort Law*. 4th edn. Clarendon Press, Oxford

McHale J, Fox M, Murphy J (1997) *Health Care Law*. Sweet and Maxwell, London

McHale J, Tingle J, Peysner J (1998) *Law and Nursing*. Butterworth Heinemann, Oxford

Montgomery J (1997) *Health Care Law*. Oxford University Press, Oxford

Pitt G (2000) *Employment Law*. 4th edn. Sweet and Maxwell, London

Rowson R (1990) *An Introduction to Ethics for Nurses*. Scutari Press, London

Skegg PDG (1998) *Law, Ethics and Medicine*. 2nd edn. Oxford University Press, Oxford

Stone J, Matthews J (1996) *Complementary Medicine and the Law*. Oxford University Press, Oxford

Tingle J, Cribb A (eds) (1995) *Nursing Law and Ethics*. Blackwell Science, Oxford

Tschudin V, Marks-Maran D (1993) *Ethics: A Primer for Nurses*. Baillière Tindall, London

White R, Carr P, Lowe N (1991) *A Guide to the Children Act 1989*. Butterworths, London

Young AP (1989) *Legal Problems in Nursing Practice*. Harper & Row, London

Young AP (1994) *Law and Professional Conduct in Nursing*. 2nd edn. Scutari Press, London

Zander M (1995) *Police and Criminal Evidence Act*. 3rd edn. Sweet and Maxwell, London

Glossary

Accusatorial	A system of court proceedings where the two sides contest the issues (contrast with inquisitorial).
Act of Parliament	Statute.
Actionable *per se*	A court action where the claimant does not have to show loss, damage or harm to obtain compensation, eg. an action for trespass to the person.
Actus reus	The essential element of a crime which must be proved to secure a conviction, as opposed to the mental state of the accused (*mens rea*).
Adversarial	The approach adopted in an accusatorial system.
Advocate	A person who pleads for another: it could be paid and professional, such as a barrister or solicitor, or it could be a lay advocate either paid or unpaid.
Assault	A threat of unlawful contact (trespass to the person).
Balance of probabilities	The standard of proof in civil proceedings.
Barrister	A lawyer qualified to take a case in court.
Battery	An unlawful touching (see trespass to the person).
Bolam Test	The test laid down by Judge McNair in the case of *Bolam* v. *Friern HMC* on the standard of care expected of a professional in cases of alleged negligence.
Burden of proof	The duty of a party to litigation to establish the facts, or in criminal proceedings the duty of the prosecution to establish both the *actus reus* and the *mens rea*.
Cause of action	The facts that entitle a person to sue.
Civil action	Proceedings brought in the civil courts.
Civil wrong	An act or omission which can be pursued in the civil courts by the person who has suffered the wrong (see torts).
Committal proceedings	Hearings before the magistrates to decide if a person should be sent for trial in the crown court.

Common law   Law derived from the decisions of judges, case law, judge made law.

Conditional fee system   A system whereby client and lawyer can agree that payment of fees is dependent upon the outcome of the court action.

Coroner   A person appointed to hold an inquiry (inquest) into a death in unexpected or unusual circumstances.

Criminal wrong   An act or omission which can be pursued in the criminal courts.

Damages   A sum of money awarded by a court as compensation for a tort or breach of contract.

Declaration   A ruling by the court, setting out the legal situation.

Dissenting judgement   A judge who disagrees with the decision of the majority of judges. The rules of precedent require judges to follow decisions of judges in previous cases, where these are binding upon them. In some circumstances it is possible to come to a different decision because the facts of the earlier case are not comparable to the case now being heard, and therefore the earlier decision can be 'distinguished'.

Ex gratia   As a matter of favour, eg. without admission of liability, of payment offered to a claimant.

Expert witness   Evidence given by a person whose general opinion based on training or experience is relevant to some of the issues in dispute.

Re F. ruling   A professional who acts in the best interests of an incompetent person who is incapable of giving consent, does not act unlawfully if he follows the accepted standard of care according to the Bolam Test.

Hierarchy   The recognised status of courts which results in lower courts following the decisions of higher courts (see precedent). Decisions of the House of Lords must be followed by all lower courts unless, they can be distinguished.

Indictment   A written accusation against a person, charging him with a serious crime, triable by jury.

Injunction   An order of the court restraining a person.

Inquisitorial	A system of justice whereby the truth is revealed by an inquiry into the facts conducted by the judge, eg. coroner's court.
Judicial review	An application to the High Court for a judicial or administrative decision to be reviewed and an appropriate order made, eg. declaration.
Litigation	Civil proceedings.
Magistrate	A person (Justice of the Peace or stipendiary magistrate) who hears summary (minor) offences or indictable offences which can be heard in the magistrates court.
Mens rea	The mental element in a crime (contrasted with *actus reus*).
Ombudsman	A Commissioner (eg. health, local Government) appointed by the Government to hear complaints.
Plaintiff	Term formerly used to describe one who brings an action in the civil courts. Now the term claimant is used.
Practice direction	Guidance issued by the head of the court to which they relate on the procedure to be followed.
Precedent	A decision which may have to be followed in a subsequent court hearing (see hierarchy).
Prima facie	At first sight, or sufficient evidence brought by one party to require the other party to provide a defence.
Privilege	In relation to evidence, being able to refuse to disclose it to the court.
Proof	Evidence which secures the establishment of a claimant's or prosecution's or defendant's case.
Prosecution	The pursuing of criminal offences in court.
Quantum	The amount of compensation, or the monetary value of a claim.
Reasonable doubt	To secure a conviction in criminal proceedings the prosecution must establish beyond reasonable doubt the guilt of the accused.
Solicitor	A lawyer who is qualified on the register held by the Law Society.
Statute law (statutory)	Law made by Acts of Parliament.

Strict liability	Liability for a criminal act where the mental element does not have to be proved; in civil proceedings liability without establishing negligence.
Subpoena	An order of the court requiring a person to appear as a witness (subpoena *ad testificandum*) or to bring records/documents (subpoena *duces tecum*).
Summary offence	A lesser offence which can only be heard by magistrates.
Tort	A civil wrong excluding breach of contract. It includes: negligence, trespass (to the person, goods or land), nuisance, breach of statutory duty and defamation.
Trespass to the person	A wrongful direct interference with another person. Harm does not have to be proved.
Ultra vires	Outside the powers given by law (eg. of a statutory body or company).
Vicarious liability	The liability of an employer for the wrongful acts of an employee committed while in the course of employment.

Appendix: Schedule 1 to the Human Rights Act 1998

Article 2 Right to Life

1.   Everyone's right to life shall be protected by law. No one shall be deprived of his life intentionally save in the execution of a sentence of a court following his conviction of a crime for which this penalty is provided by law.

2.   Deprivation of life shall not be regarded as inflicted in contravention of this Article when it results from the use of force which is no more than absolutely necessary:

(a)   in defence of any person from unlawful violence;
(b)   in order to effect a lawful arrest or to prevent the escape of a person lawfully detained;
(c)   in action lawfully taken for the purpose of quelling a riot or insurrection.

Article 3 Prohibition of torture

No one shall be subjected to torture or to inhuman or degrading treatment or punishment.

Article 4 Prohibition of slavery and forced labour

1.   No one shall be held in slavery or servitude.

2.   No one shall be required to perform forced or compulsory labour.

3.   For the purpose of this Article the term 'forced or compulsory labour' shall not include:

(a)   any work required to be done in the ordinary course of detention imposed according to the provisions of Article 5 of this Convention or during conditional release from such detention;
(b)   any service of a military character or, in case of conscientious objectors in countries where they are recognised, service exacted instead of compulsory military service;
(c)   any service exacted in case of an emergency or calamity threatening the life or well-being of the community;
(d)   any work or service which forms part of normal civic obligations.

Article 5 Right to liberty and security

1.   Everyone has the right to liberty and security of person. No one shall be deprived of his liberty save in the following cases and in accordance with a procedure prescribed by law:

(a)   the lawful detention of a person after conviction by a competent court;

(b)   the lawful arrest or detention of a person for non-compliance with the lawful order of a court or in order to secure the fulfilment of any obligation prescribed by law;

(c)   the lawful arrest or detention of a person effected for the purpose of bringing him before the competent legal authority on reasonable suspicion of having committed an offence or when it is reasonably considered necessary to prevent his committing an offence or fleeing after having done so;

(d)   the detention of a minor by lawful order for the purpose of educational supervision or his lawful detention of the purpose of bringing him before the competent legal authority;

(e)   the lawful detention of persons for the prevention of the spreading of infectious diseases, of persons of unsound mind, alcoholics or drug addicts or vagrants;

(f)   the lawful arrest or detention of a person to prevent his effecting an unauthorised entry into the country or of a person against whom action is being taken with a view to deportation or extradition.

2.   Everyone who is arrested shall be informed promptly, in a language which he understands, of the reasons for his arrest and of any charge against him.

3.   Everyone arrested or detained in accordance with the provisions of paragraph 1(c) of this Article shall be brought promptly before a judge or other officer authorised by law to exercise judicial power and shall be entitled to trial within a reasonable time or to release pending trial. Release may be conditioned by guarantees to appear for trial.

4.   Everyone who is deprived of his liberty by arrest or detention shall be entitled to take proceedings by which the lawfulness of his detention shall be decided speedily by a court and his release ordered if the detention is not lawful.

5.   Everyone who has been the victim of arrest or detention in contravention of the provisions of this Article shall have an enforceable right to compensation.

Article 6 Right to a fair trial

1.   In the determination of his civil rights and obligations or of any criminal charge against him, everyone is entitled to a fair and public hearing within a reasonable time by an independent and impartial tribunal established by law. Judgement shall be pronounced publicly but the press and public may be excluded from all or part of the trial in the interests of morals, public order or national security in a democratic society, where the interests of juveniles or the protection of the private life of the parties so require, or to the extent strictly necessary in the opinion of the court in special circumstances where publicity would prejudice the interests of justice.

2.   Everyone charged with a criminal offence shall be presumed innocent until proved guilty according to law.

3.   Everyone charged with a criminal offence has the following minimum rights:

(a)   to be informed promptly, in a language which he understands and in detail, of the nature and cause of the accusation against him;

(b)   to have adequate time and facilities for the preparation of his defence;

(c)   to defend himself in person or through legal assistance of his own choosing or, if he has not sufficient means to pay for legal assistance, to be given it free when the interests of justice so require;

(d) to examine or have examined witnesses against him and to obtain the attendance and examination of witnesses on his behalf under the same conditions as witnesses against him;

(e) to have the free assistance of an interpreter if he cannot understand or speak the language used in court.

Article 7 No punishment without law

1.   No one shall be held guilty of any criminal offence on account of any act or omission which did not constitute a criminal offence under national or international law at the time when it was committed. Nor shall a heavier penalty be imposed than the one that was applicable at the time the criminal offence was committed.

2.   This Article shall not prejudice the trial and punishment of any person for any act or omission which, at the time when it was committed, was criminal according to the general principles of law recognised by civilised nations.

Article 8 Right to respect for private and family life

1.   Everyone has the right to respect for his private and family life, his home and his correspondence.

2.   There shall be no interference by a public authority with the exercise of this right except such as is in accordance with the law and is necessary in a democratic society in the interests of national security, public safety or the economic well-being of the country, for the prevention of disorder or crime, for the protection of health or morals, or for the protection of the rights and freedoms of others.

Article 9 Freedom of thought, conscience and religion

1.   Everyone has the right to freedom of thought, conscience and religion; this right includes freedom to change his religion or belief and freedom, either alone or in community with others and in public or private, to manifest his religion or belief, in worship, teaching, practice and observance.

2.   Freedom to manifest one's religion or beliefs shall be subject only to such limitations as are prescribed by law and are necessary in a democratic society in the interests of public safety, for the protection of public order, health or morals, or for the protection of the rights and freedoms of others.

Article 10 Freedom of expression

1.   Everyone has the right to freedom of expression. This right shall include freedom to hold opinions and to receive and impart information and ideas without interference by public authority and regardless of frontiers. This Article shall not prevent States from requiring the licensing of broadcasting, television or cinema enterprises.

2.   The exercise of these freedoms, since it carries with it duties and responsibilities, may be subject to such formalities, conditions, restrictions or penalties as are prescribed by law and are necessary in a democratic society, in the interests of national security, territorial integrity or public safety, for the prevention of disorder or crime, for the protection of health or morals, for the protection of reputation or rights of others, for preventing the disclosure of information received in confidence, or for maintaining the authority and impartiality of the judiciary.

Article 11 Freedom of assembly and association

1.   Everyone has the right to freedom of peaceful assembly and to freedom of association with others, including the right to form and to join trade unions for the protection of his interests.

2.   No restrictions shall be placed on the exercise of these rights other than such as are prescribed by law and are necessary in a democratic society in the interests of national security or public safety, for the prevention of disorder or crime, for the protection of health or morals or for the protection of the rights and freedoms of others. This Article shall not prevent the imposition of lawful restrictions on the exercise of these rights by members of the armed forces, of the police or of the administration of the State.

Article 12 Right to marry

Men and women of marriageable age have the right to marry and to found a family, according to the national laws governing the exercise of this right.

Article 14 Prohibition of discrimination

The enjoyment of the rights and freedoms set forth in this Convention shall be secured without discrimination on any ground such as sex, race, colour, language, religion, political or other opinion, national or social origin, association with a national minority, property, birth or other status.

Article 16 Restrictions on political activity of aliens

Nothing in Articles 10, 11 and 14 shall be regarded as preventing the High Contracting Parties from imposing restrictions on the political activity of aliens.

Article 17 Prohibition of abuse of rights

Nothing in this Convention may be interpreted as implying for any State, group or person any right to engage in any activity or perform any act aimed at the destruction of any of the rights and freedoms set forth herein or at their limitation to a greater extent than is provided for in the Convention.

Article 18 Limitation on use of restrictions on rights

The restrictions permitted under this Convention to the said rights and freedoms shall not be applied for any purpose other than those for which they have been prescribed.

The first protocol

Article 1

Every natural or legal person is entitled to the peaceful enjoyment of his possessions. No one shall be deprived of his possessions except in the public interest and subject to the conditions provided for by law and by the general principles of international law.

The preceeding provisions shall not, however, in any way impair the right of a State to enforce such laws as it deems necessary to control the use of property in accordance with the general interest or to secure the payment of taxes or other contributions or penalties.

Article 2

No person shall be denied the right to education. In the exercise of any functions which it assumes in relation to education and to teaching, the State shall respect the right of parents to ensure such education and teaching in conformity with their own religious and philosophical convictions.

Article 3

The High Contracting Parties undertake to hold free elections at reasonable intervals by secret ballot, under conditions which will ensure the free expression of the opinion of the people in the choice of the legislature.

Index of cases

Index of Statutes

Index